Classical Formulas in the Western Herbal Tradition

P.O. Box 32
Shortsville, New York 14548
lesmoore_nd@hotmail.com
www.classicalformulas.com
www.drlesmoore.com

All rights reserved

Copyright © 2002 by Les Moore, ND, MSOM, LAc.

No part of this book may be reproduced or transmitted in any form or by any means, electronic or mechanical, including photocopying, recording, or by any information storage and retrieval system, without permission in writing from the author.

The information in this book is for educational purposes only and should not be used to diagnose and treat diseases. All serious health conditions should be treated by a competent health practitioner. Neither the publisher nor the author of this book in any way dispense medical advice, prescribe remedies, or assume responsibility for those who choose to treat themselves.

ISBN 0-9742049-0-0

PRINTED IN THE UNITED STATES OF AMERICA.

DEDICATION

This book is dedicated to my mother
Who showed me God
And to my father
Who showed me God's presence in nature.

Foreword

Herbal medicine is highly regarded and utilized in almost all cultures of the world. Particularly in China and the rest of the Orient, herbs are used to treat most diseases encountered in the clinical setting. Even today, although modern Western medicine practices have been essentially adopted in these Eastern nations, it is still very common for Medical Doctors there to refer patients who are not responding well to pharmaceutical treatments to traditional herbalists.

The fact that Eastern herbal medicine often makes up for modern Western medicine's shortcomings is no doubt attributed to the high academic standards Easterners set for herbal medicine study. In fact, the standard herbal medicine texts contain a synthesis of herbal knowledge originating from many brilliant herbalist-physicians of times long passed. It is from these texts that Eastern herbal medicine practitioners glean a tried-and-true methodology to effectively manage a vast array of health conditions today.

Dr. Moore's new book, ***Classical Formulas in the Western Herbal Tradition***, is a refreshing and much-needed first step in revitalizing the scholarship of the Western herbal medicine tradition. Similar to scholarly textbooks utilized in the East, Dr. Moore methodically presents scores of original tried-and-true herbal combinations formulated by the pioneers of the Western herbal medicine tradition. Formulae descriptions include clear explanation of actions, indications/applications, contraindications, form and dosages, as well as valuable commentary on the formula and its modifications to suit individual patients.

The publication of this book is indeed timely in the light of the ever escalating maligning herbal medicine faces in the media. Headlines appear more like a scare tactic ploy to dissuade the public from considering herbs as a health care option. Almost all are unsubstantiated single-case reports. In reality, the truth lies hidden behind these headlines.

What the media neglects to mention is that the appropriate use of *prescription* medications continues to be one of the top five leading causes of death in America today. Beyond that statistic lies an even greater number of individuals receiving medications inappropriately and whose often severe adverse drug effects go unrecognized, and – even worse- unreported.

Dr. Moore has done a great service for the medical profession with this work. He returns readers to the wisdom that brought herbal medicine to the forefront of healing in days before pharmaceuticals had taken their stronghold on modern healthcare. This text will surely serve to guide the way to the safer and more effective use of herbal medicine in the West.

Thaddeus Jacobs, N.D., L.Ac., Dipl. C.H. NCCAOM
Co-author of ***Interactions Between Drugs & Natural Medicines***
Santa Barbara, CA, July 27

ACKNOWLEDGEMENTS

This book did not manifest itself. It stands on the shoulders of giants who contributed information, ideas, concepts and corrections to this effort. In referring to giants, I mean those who composed or preserved the formulas, as well as those who lifted me up and encouraged me to continue this project.

I must first thank God, who gave us the leaves of the trees for medicine.

I thank my beautiful wife Kimberly for allowing me to look at every plant we pass by. Her love and support is invaluable. I must also thank my precious daughters, Molly and Michaela, for allowing me to teach them about every plant we see together.

I must then thank my father, who showed me the plants of the southern Appalachians and Sandhills and how to use them in the long herbal tradition that goes back through the mists of time. I must thank my mother, who then showed me how to give the herbs with care and compassion.

I would like to thank Dr. Jim Horton for showing me field botany and Dr. Dan Petillo for teaching amazing classes in dendrology at Western Carolina University. Thanks to Dr. Lawrence Kolenbrander for putting these natural resources into perspective. Thanks to Ron Huff for contributing all of that "dirt" time with me in the mountains of North Carolina.

Thanks to Mary Chiltoskey and Walt Burchett for helping preserve the Cherokee herbal medicine.

I must thank Cascade Anderson-Geller for sharing her love of herbalism and Sharleen Andrews-Miller and Judy Bluehorse for their love of herbs and herbal medicine making.

Those who have taught me Naturopathic Medicine are too numerous to mention, but I must thank those who shared their great knowledge of botanical medicine with me:

Jill Stansbury, ND, for her grace, music, art and intelligence about herbal medicine, pharmacognosy, and pharmacology.

Bill Mitchell, ND, for preserving the past and prospecting into the future.

Francis Brinker, ND, for putting such great ideas about herbal medicine onto paper.

Wade Boyle, ND, for preserving some of our heritage of botanical medicine.

Friedhelm Kirchfeld, for creating the greatest Naturopathic library in the world at the National College of Naturopathic Medicine.

Jared Zeff, ND, LAc., for offering a philosophical base in which to apply Naturopathic botanical medicine in the context of Naturopathy.

Steven Baily, ND, for keeping the Nature Cure in Naturopathy.

Chris Meletis, ND, for sharing natural pharmacology and his natural pharmacy.

Ed Alstat, ND, for preserving the Eclectic ideas and the heritage of herbal medicine.

Thad Jacobs, ND, MSOM, LAc., for allowing me to share and exchange ideas.

Steve Marsden, DVM, ND, MSOM, LAc, for those discussions in herbal energetics.

Josh Berry, ND, for those herbal forays into the Pacific Northwest.

Durr Elmore, DC, ND, DHANP, for detailing the finer points of the homeopathic indications of the materia medica.

Prem Dev, ND, for pulling together three generations of healing and mastering the materia medica.

Michael Murray, ND, for reaching so many people through his books and inspiring me to start Naturopathic medical school.

Dohn Kruschwitz, MD, ND, for showing me how to think critically through a clinical problem.

Jack Daugherty, DC, ND, for showing me how to use my intuition with herbs in a better manner.

Stephen Sporn, ND, for helping preserve the history of Naturopathy so we can try to avoid making the same mistakes twice, and for his fire for Naturopathy.

John Collins, ND, DHANP, for showing me how to take a thorough history.

Tori Hudson, ND, for sharing her knowledge of the use of herbs in gynecology.

From my study of Classical Chinese Medicine I must thank:

Heiner Fruehauf, PhD., LAc, who stepped right out of the Han Dynasty and brought us healing as practiced for centuries.

Jim Cleaver, LAc, who showed me how to strive for perfection in understanding single herbs and pairs.

Dr. Rihui Long, for transmitting to me the Shang Han Lun and the concepts of the Spleen Tonifying school.

Dr. Mengke Kou, who transmitted to me deep caring and the concepts of the Kidney Tonifying school.

Dr. Haosheng Zhang, who told me to always return to the classics and basic theory, and taught me the intricacies of the Wenbing School of Herbal Medicine.

Dr. Michael Chang, who taught a great formulas modification class.

Dr. Liu, for preserving the Wenbing school in English.

Dr. Zeng, for showing me some of the nuances of the pulse.

David Frierman, LAc. for showing me how to really care for people.

From the great tradition of Ayurveda I would like to thank:

Professor R.H. Singh, for sharing the details of Pancha Karma.

Dr. Frank Ros, for sharing Ayurveda and marmapuncture.

Dr. Vasant Lad, for sharing his herbal knowledge and Ayurveda.

I would also like to thank:

Paul Bergner, for preserving herbal medicine through *Medical Herbalism* and allowing me to share and exchange ideas with him.

7 Song, for allowing me to teach these ideas at the Northeast School of Botanical Medicine.

Clifton Springs Hospital and Clinic, for preserving the health of many people and the medicine of the people, and especially to Charlotte Wytias and Gladys Simons for helping to make The Springs of Clifton such a wonderful healing center.

New York Chiropractic College, for its vision of integrated healthcare.

Carol Collie, for assisting in the proofing of this book.

Dan Inosanto, for teaching me how to transfer knowledge.

I must also thank Michele Wilbur, Master Herbalist, Master Chef, and Nutritionist for her great help in editing this book.

A great, big thanks to all of my patients who have shown me how these herbs really work.

And a big thanks to Bonnie Hayman for her love of natural medicine and great editorial skills and for pulling this book together.

May all of your dreams come true!

Table of Contents

Preface

The purpose of this book is to provide a clinical and academic handbook for the use of herbal formulas in the clinic and a systematic and scholarly study in the classroom. We have many great texts and handbooks examining the use of single herbs, their functions and properties, their pharmacology, and their interactions with drugs, nutrients, and other herbs. What is missing is a book that can take these herbs and put them into formulas that have stood the test of time and classify them in holistic, useful ways. Herbs have been the norm of medicine for at least the last six thousand years. For most of the cultures and systems of medicine, the use of single herbs, or simpling, has been used by the people (lay practitioners, home remedies) and the use of formulas has been practiced by the physicians, or those formally trained in a particular system of therapeutic herbalism. Single herbs can be powerful agents of healing, but herbal formulas can act synergistically and be tailored and modified for each and every unique patient, even changing as the patient or environment changes.

Les Moore ND, MSOM, LAc
The Springs of Clifton
Clifton Springs Hospital
Clifton Springs, New York
July 2002

lesmoore_nd@hotmail.com
www.classicalformulas.com
www.drlesmoore.com

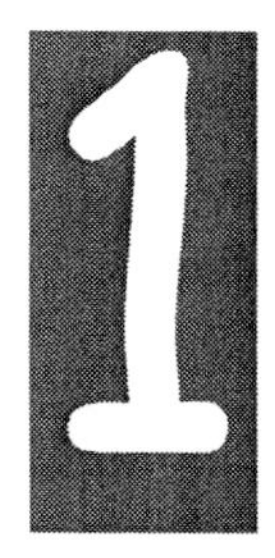

Introduction

I began this book by looking at classical western herbal formulas through the lens of Chinese herbal medicine. Just as people can learn more about their native language by studying a foreign language, so can they learn more about their indigenous system of herbal therapeutics by studying a different system. This is what happened as I studied classical Chinese herbal medicine. At first I noticed similarities, then, after studying more, I noticed great differences. Later, I again saw the similarities and realized that we were just looking at the plants from a different perspective.

During my study of classical Chinese medicine, I found myself reading the Shang Han Lun by Zhang Zhongjing. In the preface to this 2000 year old Chinese medical classic, Dr. Zhang Zhongjing states:

> "...I don't quite understand why scholars today do not pay more attention to these formulas and techniques when treating their elders, healing the poor, and maintaining their own health. They do little but vie for fame and power and delight themselves with improving their physical appearance while neglecting their spiritual development. If one has no skin, how can there be any hair? During a serious epidemic, victims of the disease become terrified and do not know what to do. Under present circumstances they must submit themselves to the care of witch doctors or depend upon divine providence in the hope of prolonging their lives. Alas! It is a foolish world that indulges itself in the acquisition of fame and wealth and regards life so lightly. Is this the true meaning of glory and power? People who compete for superficial success without caring for the essentials, who are indifferent to bodily care and indulge only in material gain, are as much in danger as though walking on an icy bridge abutting a valley. One who fails to learn how to love both others and oneself is not unlike a homeless wandering spirit seeking transitory worldly pleasures.

> During the first ten years of the Chien-an era (A.D. 196) of the Later Han dynasty, two-thirds of my relatives (more than two hundred) succumbed to disease, seven-tenths of which (deaths) were due to an epidemic fever. For this reason and in consideration of all those lost and not saved in the past, I decided to seek diligently ancient instructions and try to adopt for use various well-known formulas (Hsu,1981)."

I find myself today sitting in the same place as Dr. Zhang Zhongjing nearly 2000 years ago. In the name of science we throw the baby out with the bath water, discarding treatments that worked for centuries, losing entire schools of thought, for the hope of some hollow promise that was discovered yesterday or to meet the needs of some broken socio-politico-economic system of healthcare that is not oriented toward the people.

We must remember that 'science' means 'to know.' There are many ways of knowing, some that we may never understand. The modern scientific method is only one way of knowing, and is based on a very reductionist model. Some models of knowing are very holistic, and can complement a reductionist approach. Today's science will be tomorrow's misunderstanding, because we will never entirely know the whole picture. Science is only our attempt to understand the phenomena that happens around us. With all of our science, anatomy, physiology, biochemistry, diagnostic imaging, and laboratory science, what we *know* about the human body is a drop in the ocean compared to what *is* the human body. Empirical, historical, anthropological, and ethnobotanical knowledge can help us understand how to approach the human and healing.

I was first trained by my father in the herbal tradition of the Southern Appalachian bioregion. This lineage is passed along orally with its foundation in the Native American herbal tradition (particularly Cherokee), the Colonial American Folk tradition, and in Thomsonian herbalism. This tradition consists mainly of simpling, requiring an intimate knowledge of plants and their habitats, some small herbal combinations or pairs, and a few composite formulas. This knowledge later sparked the desire that led me to Naturopathic medical school, where I would learn herbalism in the Naturopathic Botanical Medicine tradition, which has a very broad base and eclectic background. These systems are thorough, and they have helped and still help millions of people, but I felt drawn to also learn herbalism from the classical Chinese tradition.

I was enamored and in awe of Chinese herbal medicine as soon as I started studying it formally. Maybe it was the exoticism, but I believe it was the discipline, the scholarly tradition, and the clinical effectiveness that pulled me in. The discipline was evident in the professors' mastery of the extensive Chinese materia medica and in the complexity of the study of classical Chinese herbal formulas and modifications. After five years of medical school, I believe there is no subject as complex and difficult in any medical school. The clinical effectiveness was totally astounding. Here were physicians who had at their disposal all of the armamentarium of modern medical science, but chose to use only herbal formulas in the treatment of their patients, with extremely successful results. These formulas were not only effective in acute diseases, but unbelievably effective in the treatment of difficult and recalcitrant diseases. What really struck me the most, and is the subject of this book, is the long, scholarly tradition of studying and applying the formulas. The herbs and formulas are studied in a classical manner with the same intensity and fervor as a seminary theologian studying scripture. In fact, studying Chinese medicine according to the classics reminds me of Biblical exegesis, where one goes to unfathomable depths to find what the original meaning of the word or character is, and attempts to apply that to life today.

This scholarly tradition I found missing in Western herbal medicine. Of course, there are ancient texts and formulas, but these are quickly lost, along with whole schools of thought, in the name of modern science. Newly acquired knowledge is good, but one shouldn't throw the baby out with the bath water. What the ancients practiced was effective, and what practitioners have practiced in the past few centuries is still as effective today as it was in the past. Knowing that Western herbal medicine is effective, and has been practiced extensively in the past, I went searching for this scholarly tradition.

What I found was that the scholarly tradition was sparse, and mostly in the past. Nothing was really done to bring the schools of thought together. Neither was there a scholarly tradition of studying the formulas or of even organizing the formulas. There had been plenty written and discussed about single remedies, but most practitioners applied formulas. These weren't being taught in the schools, and if they were, it was just from one school of thought. Most formulas being used were made up by the practitioner without using any foundation, no body of knowledge to build upon. This was different than what the Chinese were doing. They were learning the single herbs in detail, including the energetics (which we had long stopped using), then the herbal pairs and their functions, then the formulas as have been applied through the ages, and finally individual modification of these ancient formulas to meet the patients' specific needs. This had been practiced in the past in Western herbal medicine, but had been essentially lost to modern medical science.

What I attempt to do in this book is examine classical formulas in the Western herbal tradition. Due to the amount of research that is available on Western formulas, 'classical' is defined in this book as a formula that has been used successfully by more than one generation or has shown up in at least two texts that are at least one generation apart. 'Western' refers mainly to Europe and North America. 'Formulas' refers to an herbal composite of two or more herbs used therapeutically.

The Western Herbal Tradition

Herbal medicine in the West has produced numerous schools of thought. Most are somewhat similar in structure, but they can vary extremely. Naturopathic botanical medicine has drawn from most of the schools of the Western tradition. America has been a melting pot of peoples and cultures, and has also been a melting pot of herbal medicine traditions. The herbal medicine that is forming now not only incorporates much of the Western herbal tradition, but also includes both Chinese and Ayurvedic herbal medicine and the emerging pharmacopoeias of the rain forest and other peoples.

The history of Western herbal medicine is rich and varied. Its roots reach back into the mists of time and its branches leap forward to a time now when single constituents can be isolated and studied to gather a fuller understanding of a plant's potential. Today's practitioner must look retrospectively into the past to uncover treasures that can be applied successfully today and simultaneously be prospecting into the future for clinical gems.

This book focuses on the classical approach to Western herbal medicine, and a study of the historical aspects of Western herbalism is necessary for a scholarly study. A fuller study of the history of Western herbalism can be found in Barbara Griggs ***Green Pharmacy: The History and Evolution of Western Herbal Medicine***. It is an excellent book, even though her understanding of the depth of botanical medicine training received in American Naturopathic Medical schools is lacking.

Western herbal medicine draws its traditions from Europe and the Americas. Many of the herbs that are used now and were used centuries ago come from both the Near and Far East. A sharing of knowledge and a penchant for practicality has always led western systems to a functional approach, and herbal medicine is no exception. We have roots that lead back to Hippocrates, Galen, Pythagoras, Dioscorides, Paracelsus, Hildegard von Bingen, Culpeper, and many others. In the last two centuries herbal medicine has grown by leaps and bounds. The Europeans were starting to mix their understanding of herbs with the Native Americans. Thomsonian herbalism was founded by Samuel Thomson in the early nineteenth century. This quickly spread back to England via Albert Coffin. Eclectic herbalism later was formed, and Physio-medicalism evolved out of Thomsonian herbalism. These schools of thought later merged into Naturopathic botanical medicine and medical herbalism.

The Formulas

The formulas represented here are only a beginning. A beginning in that there are many more formulas to classify and some of these probably need to be reclassified into categories that better fit them, and a beginning in that this work, to be truly scholarly, should be scrutinized by the herbal community at large.

Each formula is broken down into ten sections, allowing one to study the formula in a handy fashion. Most of what I have tried to do is of a historical manner, to preserve the way the formula was originally presented and the way it was originally thought to function. I have made some huge leaps in interpretation, though. Most of these leaps come from the Chinese perspective regarding the way a formula functions. This transfer of knowledge was difficult, but I believe necessary to more fully understand these formulas and what they can do for patients.

The first great leap deals with categorizing these herbal formulas. Some have never been categorized the way they are here, but have been done so because of their function. Physiological actions upon the body are similar no matter what therapeutic herbal system one has learned (an emetic action is the same in Chinese, Cherokee, Physio-medical, etc. herbal systems). The way the Chinese view a formula from a holistic perspective is the reason they have been categorized the way they are.

The second great leap I have made is the assigning of confirmatory pulse and tongue pictures to the formulas. Some pulse and tongue pictures have been assigned to the formulas already, some come from herbal remedies that make up the formula, some come from the symptom complex described within the school of thought of the formula, but most come from outside the particular school. This leap was made when a symptom complex was the same in a sister Chinese formula, and the actions, functions, and properties of the formulas were the same or similar.

How to Use This Book

Each formula is broken down into ten sections, examining the therapeutic principles, constituents, form, dosage, indications, applications, contraindications, herbs and actions, modifications, and a brief commentary. The Therapeutic Principle section attempts to understand the major focus and function of the herbal formula. The Constituents section tries to record the original herbs and amounts used in the preparation of the basic formula. The Form section attempts to record in which form the formula was used, or its vehicle of delivery. The Dosage section gives a dosage that was recommended by the formulator or that later was accepted as the appropriate dosage for an adult. The Indication section lists signs and symptoms that can lead one to this formula. The Application section lists when this formula can be used. The Contraindication section lists any contraindications that are known. The Herbs and Actions section attempts to show the functions of herbs and herb pairs in the formula. The Modification section demonstrates some modifications to the formula that can help guide it properly to the patient. The Commentary section discusses outstanding or historical aspects of the formula.

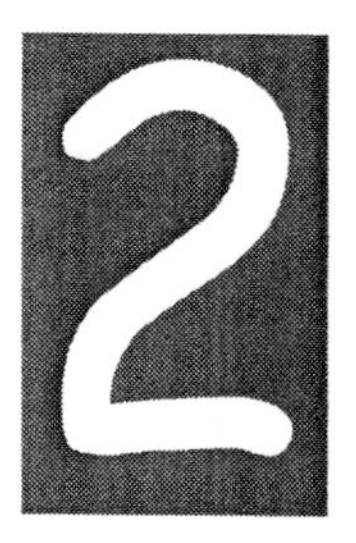

The Diaphoretics

Use

- To induce perspiration and modify the body temperature.
- To relieve upper respiratory tract infections and acute infectious disease.
- To dilate peripheral capillaries.
- If you require herbs that are febrifugal, antiviral, and antibacterial.

Formulas

Jethro Kloss' Composition Powder

Therapeutic Principle
Diaphoretic with a pungent and warm nature.

Constituents
- 4 ounces Bayberry (*Myrica cerifera*)
- 2 ounces Ginger (*Zingiber officinale*)
- 1 ounce White Pine (*Pinus strobus*)
- 1 dram Cloves (*Syzygium aromaticum*)
- 1 dram Cayenne (*Capsicum frutescens*)

Form
Powder.

Dosage
One cup of tea every hour until the patient perspires freely. To prepare, use all of the herbs in powdered form, mix and put through a fine sieve twice. Steep one teaspoonful in a covered cup of boiling water for fifteen minutes. Drink the clear liquid poured off from the sediment (Kloss, 1939).

Indication
Fever, hoarseness, lack of perspiration, cramps, colic, rhinitis, pharyngitis, body aches, sluggish circulation, cough, headache, intolerance of cold, no perspiration. The pulse tends to be superficial and tight, while the tongue usually has a thin white coating.

Application
Colds, influenza, fever, laryngitis, pharyngitis, rhinitis, cough, asthma.

Contraindication
Contraindicated in fever with perspiration.

Herbs and Actions
The Ginger, Cayenne, and Bayberry are stimulating and diaphoretic. The Ginger is pungent. The Cloves act with the Ginger and Bayberry as aromatics, opening the pores and the orifices of the head. The White Pine acts as an expectorant, demulcent, and diuretic, benefiting the kidneys and helping to eliminate toxins.

Modification
For severe cough, add Tussilago and Verbascum. With perspiration, remove Cayenne and Ginger. To make Thomson's Composition Powder, remove the Pine and add Hemlock. This acts as a stimulating alterative and a sialogogue, for dry mouth and throat, and also for difficulty breathing (Grieves, 1931).

COMMENTARY

This formula from Jethro Kloss has been a tried and proven remedy. It will clear the body of a cold and bring a fever down. It is a modification of Samuel Thomson's Composition Powder, which has been used effectively for a couple of centuries. Samuel Thomson's Composition Powder has the addition of Hemlock and the deletion of the Pine. This guides the formula more in the direction of a stimulating alterative.

Potter's Diaphoretic

THERAPEUTIC PRINCIPLE

Diaphoretic with a cool nature.

CONSTITUENTS

- 8 parts Marshmallow root (*Althea officinalis*)
- 4 parts Licorice (*Glycyrrhiza glabra*)
- 4 parts Spanish iris (*Iris florentina*)
- 4 parts Ground ivy (*Glechoma hederacea*)
- 1 part Aniseed (*Pimpinella anisum*)
- 4 parts Coltsfoot leaves (*Tussilago farfara*)
- 2 parts Red poppy flowers (*Papaver somniferum*)
- 2 parts Mullein (*Verbascum thapsus*)

FORM

Tea.

DOSAGE

Mix and use one teaspoonful of herbs to each cup of boiling water, simmer fifteen minutes, then steep and set aside until cool enough to drink. Use one-half cup or more every two hours, or more frequently if needed.

INDICATION

Indicated for the common cold with cough, fever, and a slight thirst. The pulse tends to be superficial and rapid, while the tongue usually has a thin white coating. There is no perspiration present. (Usually for the initial stage of the cold.)

Application
Common cold, influenza, acute bronchitis, acute tonsillitis, cough.

Contraindication
Contraindicated with signs and symptoms of extreme cold and chilliness.

Herbs and Actions
Althea acts as a demulcent, emollient, and diuretic. The Mullein and Coltsfoot act as demulcents and expectorants. The Poppy is cooling and acts as an expectorant and diaphoretic. Aniseed acts as a carminative, stimulant, and pectoral. Ground Ivy is cooling and acts as a tonic and diuretic. The Orris root directs the formula toward the lungs.

Modifications
Add Self-heal Spike for conjunctivitis or epidemic conjunctivitis. Add Peppermint with more signs of sore throat.

Commentary
This formula first appeared with Samuel Potter, and later was recorded by Dr. Christopher. As the patient is using the tea, keep him or her well covered with a hot water bottle on the feet and a vinegar soaked towel surrounding the feet.

Sweat-Inducing Tea

Therapeutic Principle
Diaphoretic with a pungent and cooling nature.

Constituents
- 1 part Linden flowers (*Tilia europea*)
- 1 part Elder blossoms (*Sambucus nigra*)
- 1 part Mullein flowers (*Verbascum phlomoides*)
- 1 part Peppermint (*Mentha piperita*)

Form
Tea.

Dosage
Mix equal parts, pour one cup boiling water over one to two teaspoons of herb, let steep for ten minutes, strain, stir in one to two teaspoons of honey, drink hot.

Indication
Symptoms of common cold: aching, runny nose, headache, cough, mucus in chest, sore throat, irritability. The pulse tends to be superficial and the tongue usually has a white coat.

Application
Common cold, influenza, cough, sinusitis, earache, sore throat, bronchitis, infections.

Contraindication
Contraindicated in cases of extreme chilliness.

Herbs and Actions
The Linden and Elder act as diaphoretics. The Elder and Mullein loosen phlegm. The Linden promotes sputum formation while the Mullein alleviates a tickling cough. The Peppermint stimulates, invigorates the stomach, clears up breathing, and soothes a sore throat (Rauch, 1967).

Modification
For hayfever or asthma, add Grindelia. For paroxysmal laryngeal cough, add Trifolium. With dry, hot skin, add Achillea and Pulsatilla. With chronic sinusitis, add Pulsatilla. For weakening night sweats, add Salvia (Priest, 1982).

COMMENTARY

This is an old naturopathic formula from the European tradition. It appears in Erich Rauch's book, ***Naturopathic Treatment of Colds and Infectious Diseases***. It was probably influenced by Dr. Rauch's mentor, Dr. Brauchle. Dr. Rauch used a lot of nature cure treatments with his herbalism. He was fond of giving enemas, baths, steams, hot packs, and other hydrotherapeutic treatments to enhance the effectiveness of herbal medicine.

Sudorific Powders

THERAPEUTIC PRINCIPLE

Diaphoretic with pungent and cool nature.

CONSTITUENTS

- 4 ounces Lobelia (*Lobelia inflata*)
- 4 ounces Pleurisy root (*Asclepias tuberosa*)
- 4 ounces Skunk Cabbage (*Symplocarpus foetidus*)
- 4 ounces Crawley root or Feverroot (*Pterospora andromedea*)

FORM

Powder.

DOSAGE

One quarter of a teaspoonful every hour, until a gentle perspiration is produced (Colby, 1846).

INDICATION

Cough, fever with no perspiration, intolerance of cold, general aching, headache. The pulse tends to be superficial and tight, while the tongue usually has a thin white coating.

APPLICATION

Cough, common cold, influenza, typhus, scarlet fever.

CONTRAINDICATION

Contraindicated with a fever with perspiration, contraindicated in pregnancy.

HERBS AND ACTIONS

Lobelia acts as a stimulant relaxant, diaphoretic and expectorant. Asclepias acts as an expectorant and influences blood flow to the surface. Feverroot acts as a diaphoretic and febrifuge. Skunk Cabbage acts as a diaphoretic, expectorant, and diuretic.

MODIFICATION

With bronchitis, pleurisy, or peritonitis, add Zingiber. With pneumonia, add Dioscorea and Zingiber. With influenza, add Solidago and Zingiber (Priest, 1982).

COMMENTARY

This formula is from Samuel Thomson, and recorded by Benjamin Colby in ***A Guide to Health*** in 1846. The dosage was increased when used in typhus or scarlet fever. The formula was considered "Valuable for producing perspiration and equalizing the circulation; highly useful for a cough, and admirably adapted to break up a cold (Colby, 1846)."

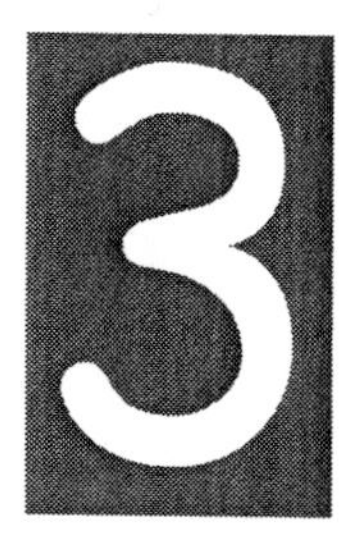

The Antipyretics

Use

- To decrease fever.
- To reduce fever symptoms such as red face, constipation, inflammation, abscess.
- To increase immune system activity.
- If you require herbs that are usually cooling in nature.
- If you require herbs that are usually antiviral, antibacterial, antifungal.

Formulas

Fever Compound

Therapeutic Principle
Eliminate heat and fever.

Constituents
- 1 ounce Catnip, powder (*Nepeta cataria*)
- 1 ounce Pleurisy root, powder (*Asclepias tuberosa*)
- 1 ounce Lobelia, powder (*Lobelia inflata*)
- ½ ounce Composition powder

Form
Powdered tea.

Dosage

Place one teaspoonful in one cup of boiling water, cover and steep a few minutes, sweeten to taste. Drink ¼ cup every 1½ -2 hours.

Indication

For high fever, irritability, headache, dry mouth, thirsty, amber urine, cough, red face, heat sensation in the face and chest. The pulse tends to be rapid and sometimes forceful, the tongue usually appears red, sometimes with a yellow coating.

Application

Fever, pneumonia, infection, acute urinary tract infection, infection of the oral cavity, septicemia.

Contraindication

Contraindicated in pregnancy.

Herbs and Actions

Catnip acts as a diaphoretic and a refrigerant. Composition Powder acts as a diaphoretic. Asclepias acts as a peripheral and capillary relaxant and autonomic stimulant. Lobelia acts as a diaphoretic and general systemic relaxant with diffusive stimulation.

Modification

In case of depressed or low vitality, add Virginia snake root (*Aristolochia serpentaria*) or Canada snake root (*Asarum canadense*). As a diffusive stimulant, add Ginger (*Zingiber officinale*) to intensify the therapeutic action of catnip. With pneumonia, add Dioscorea. With influenza, add Solidago. With restlessness and nervous irritation, add Chamomile (Priest, 1982).

Commentary

This formula was recorded by Dr. Christopher (1976) in ***School of Natural Healing.*** It demonstrates the use of Composition Powder, a much older formula, as a driving force in the construction of another formula. The Composition Powder, as a whole, acts as another herb within the formula.

Fever Formula

Therapeutic Principle
Eliminate heat and toxins.

Constituents
- ½ ounce Hyssop (*Hyssopus officinalis*)
- ½ ounce Vervain (*Verbena officinalis*)
- ½ ounce Raspberry leaves (*Rubus ideaus*)
- ½ ounce Centuary (*Erythraea centaurium*)
- 1 teaspoonful Cayenne (*Capsicum minimum*)

Form
Tea.

Dosage
One teaspoonful, warm, every hour. To prepare, simmer the first four herbs in one quart of water for 20 minutes, then strain hot over the cayenne.

Indication
Fever, thirst, sore throat, dry mouth, dry skin, headache, dark urine, irritability. The pulse tends to be rapid, maybe superficial, and the tongue usually appears red.

Application
Fever, tonsillitis, throat inflammation, herpes infection, urinary tract infection.

Contraindication
Contraindicated in fever with perspiration and in pregnancy.

Herbs and Actions

The herbs act as a diaphoretic to open the pores and to equalize circulation. The Raspberry leaves and Cayenne are the febrifuges in the formula. Cayenne itself brings heat to eliminate heat. Hyssop and Vervain are diuretics; Vervain also acts as a relaxant. Centaury is a powerful tonic.

Modification

Add Peppermint and Honeysuckle Flower if more intense sore throat. If throat has extreme inflammation, add violet. For whooping cough, remove Vervain, Cayenne, and Centuary, and add Turkey rhubarb, Bayberry bark, and Thyme.

Commentary

This formula appeared with Dr. Christopher, and is to be administered with a foot wrap of cloth wrung out in apple cider vinegar and kept warm with a hot water bottle. Dr. Christopher was trained as a Master Herbalist through Dominion Herbal College in Canada, and as a Naturopath in the United States. He literally reached thousands of people with his seminars and books, helping to pass on the tradition of Thomsonian herbalism and Physio-Medicalism.

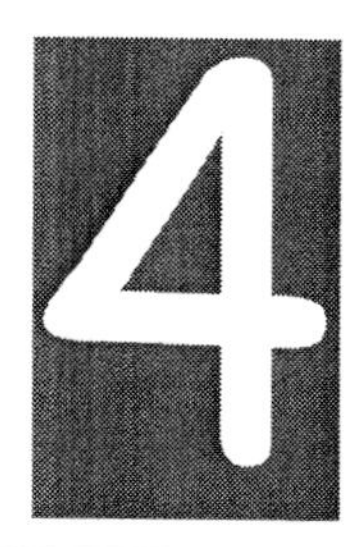

The Regulating Formulas

Use

- To regulate the organ systems.
- If you require an herb to have an alterative effect.
- To relieve stagnation within a particular organ or organ system.
- To harmonize and balance function and metabolism.

Formulas

Robert's Formula

Therapeutic Principle

Regulate the stomach.

Constituents

- 1 part Goldenseal (*Hydrastis canadensis*)
- 1 part Echinacea (*Echinacea angustifolium*)
- 1 part Marshmallow (*Althea officinalis*)
- 1 part Poke root (*Phytolacca americana*)
- 1 part Geranium (*Geranium maculatum*)

Form

Tincture or capsules.

DOSAGE:

Tincture: Ten drops four times daily before meals and before going to bed. Capsule: 2 "00" capsules four times daily before meals and before going to bed.

INDICATION:

Abdominal pain, pale facial color, fatigue, spontaneous perspiration, dyspnea, fullness sensation in the epigastric region of abdomen, loss of appetite, fullness and oppression in the chest, hiccoughs, belching, upper and lower gastrointestinal bleeding. The pulse tends to be deep and slow, while the tongue usually appears pale or light with a white coating.

APPLICATION

Gastric ulcer, duodenal ulcer, gastroenteritis, vomiting, chronic colitis, anemia, gastrectasis, ulcerative colitis, chrohn's disease, irritable bowel syndrome.

CONTRAINDICATION

Contraindicated in pregnancy.

HERBS AND ACTIONS

The Echinacea and the Poke root both work as anti-microbial and alteratives in this formula. Goldenseal is a powerful tonic, particularly towards mucus membranes. The Geranium acts as an astringent. The Marshmallow is the demulcent in the formùla; it is soothing to mucus membranes (Hoffman, 1983).

MODIFICATION

If hemorrhaging, add two parts Geranium. If painful, add Okra or Slippery elm. If a chronic ulcer, add Ginger, Baptisia, duodenal substance, Niacin, Okra, and Slippery elm, which makes Bastyr's formula. With signs of coldness, add Cinnamon and Ginger.

Commentary

This formula has two stories for the origin of its name. The first one is a sailor named Robert would go from port to port finding out the most popular ulcer remedy of the local people. From these herbs, he developed this very useful ulcer formula, Robert's Formula. The other story attributes the name to the use of Geranium in the formula, which is commonly called Herb Robert. This is a very popular formula among clinical herbalists and naturopaths. It is used mainly for ulcers, but since it is loaded with alterative herbs, it has a much wider application for gastrointestinal health (Boyle, 1993).

Dr. Carroll's Liver Formula

Therapeutic Principle

Regulate the Liver.

Constituents

- 2 parts Fringe Tree Bark (*Chionanthus virginicus*)
- 2 parts Celandine (*Chelidonium majus*)
- 1 part Mandrake (*Podophyllum peltatum*)

Form

Tincture.

Dosage

10 drops in one-half glass of water two to three times per day.

Indication

Sluggish hepatic function, indigestion, pain in the sub-costal region, mental depression, moodiness, hypochondriac distension and pain, chest fullness, belching, constipation, jaundice, decreased urination, thirst. The pulse is usually wiry and taut, but can be rapid and forceful. The tongue usually has a white or yellow greasy coating.

APPLICATION
Hepatitis, gallstones, indigestion, intestinal putrefication, eczema, jaundice, hypochondriac pain, hypertension, dysmenorrhea, irregular menstruation, breast distension, cholecystitis, cholelithiasis, depression.

CONTRAINDICATION
Contraindicated in pregnancy, impacted bile duct, and intestinal obstruction (Sherman, 1993).

HERBS AND ACTIONS
Chelidonium is an active cholagogue with influence on the liver, spleen, gallbladder, pancreas, and mesenteric lymphatic system. It acts as an alterative and a demulcent (Priest, 1982). Chionanthus is a relaxing and stimulating hepatic, alterative, cholagogue, tonic, and diuretic. It stimulates the discharge of bile and promotes the digestion of fats (Priest, 1982). Podophyllum is a hepatic tonic, alterative, and cholagogue.

MODIFICATION
With duodenal catarrh, gallstones, hepatic torpor, or catarrhal jaundice, add Berberis (Priest, 1982). With rectal prolapse or hemorrhoids, use Collinsonia (Priest, 1982). With skin eruptions, use Berberis or Arctium. With severe abdominal pain, add Corydalis. With bitter mouth, add Berberis or Goldenseal.

COMMENTARY
This was a common alcoholic extract used by Dr. O.G. Carroll (1879-1962), a turn-of-the-century naturopath and the founder of constitutional hydrotherapy. His influence was from Father Kneipp's herbalism and Thomsonian herbalism (Boyle, 1988). This is a common formula used by Naturopaths in the treatment of many liver diseases.

Dr. Shook's Liver and Jaundice Compound

Therapeutic Principle
Regulate the liver.

Constituents
- 50 grains Turkey Rhubarb root, solid extract (*Rheum palmatum*)
- 60 grains Aloe leaf, solid extract (*Aloe vera*)
- 40 grains Fringetree, solid extract (*Chioanthus virginicus*)
- 20 grains Culver's root, solid extract (*Leptandra virginica*)
- 10 grains Wahoo bark, solid extract (*Euonymus atropurpureus*)
- 10 grains Poke root, solid extract (*Phytolacca americana*)
- 2 grains Nux vomica seeds, solid extract, (*Strychnos nux vomica*)

Form
Solid extract, powdered.

Dosage
Take one to two capsules one or two times per day, according to the laxative action required. To prepare, mix thoroughly, using finely powdered material. Pass through a small-meshed sieve, and fill into approximately forty capsules (Christopher, 1976).

Indication
Biliousness, sluggish liver, constipation, dizziness, headache, nausea, abdominal fullness and bloating, decreased urination, eyes and skin color icteric, abdominal distension, belching, indigestion, moodiness, depression. The pulse tends to be wiry and taut. The tongue usually has a thin white coat.

APPLICATION

Hepatitis, headache, nausea, constipation, dysmenorrhea, irregular menstruation, catarrh of the stomach, catarrh of the gallbladder.

CONTRAINDICATION

Contraindicated in pregnancy and diarrhea.

HERBS AND ACTIONS

Rhubarb is used as a purgative, hepatic, and cholagogue, being tonic to the stomach, liver, and gallbladder. Phytolacca is used as a stimulating and relaxing alterative, promoting the removal of catabolic waste and the products of fatty degeneration. It also removes any congestion in the mesenteric lymphatic system. Fringetree acts as a relaxing and stimulating hepatic and alterative, promoting digestion of fats and stimulating the release of bile (Priest, 1982). Wahoo acts as a cholagogue, alterative, digestant, and tonic. Aloe is a laxative and purgative. Nux vomica acts as a synergist, harmonizing the other herb functions; it also works as a stomachic and tonic.

MODIFICATION

For nausea and vomiting, add Spearmint, Cinnamon, and Cloves. For severe abdominal pain, add Corydalis. With gallstones or catarrh, add Oregon Grape Root. For skin eruptions, add alteratives, such as Arctium and Rumex. With functional dyspepsia, add Goldenseal (Priest, 1982).

COMMENTARY

This formula is from Dr. Shook, recorded by Dr. Christopher (1976). It is a good example of using toxic botanicals in the correct doses and correct combinations to produce a good overall effect. It also demonstrates the Naturopathic principle of 'cleaning up the terrain' by using the purgatives to move the vital energy downward and clean up the organs.

Clymer's Liver Formulas

Therapeutic Principle

Tonify the liver.

Constituents

- 8 to 10 drops Goldenseal (*Hydrastis canadensis*)
- 4 to 8 drops Fringe Tree (*Chionanthus virginicus*)
- 5 to 8 drops Yellow Gentian (*Gentiana lutea*)
- Sufficient amount for proper elimination of Cascara Sagrada (*Rhamnus purshiana*)

Form

Tincture.

Dosage

Take the above amounts in water after each meal. Bile salts should also be taken.

Indication

Liver pain, dyspepsia, pain underneath the rib cage, bloating, liver hard to palpation, yellow skin, colic. The pulse can be wiry. The tongue can appear dark or purple.

Application

Cirrhosis, liver congestion, pain in the hypochondrium, subcostal pain, alcoholism, gallstones, hepatitis.

Herbs and Actions

Goldenseal acts as a tonic. Fringe Tree acts as a cholagogue and hepatic. Yellow Gentian acts as a bitter tonic, stomachic, and hepatic. Cascara sagrada acts as a bitter tonic and hepatic.

MODIFICATIONS

For spleen involvement, remove Gentian and Cascara, and add Redroot and Barberry. For engorgement, add Bitter Root and Dandelion to Goldenseal and remove the other herbs. For acute inflammation, just use Fringe Tree, Redroot, and Bitter Root. For a torpid liver, use Barberry, Gentian, Goldenseal, and Bitter Wood.

COMMENTARY

This formula progression comes from R. Swinburne Clymer, MD. He wrote a great book, ***Nature's Healing Agents*** (1963), which is full of clinical formulas. He founded the Natura system of medicine, which uses the herbal healing agents considered most natural from the Thomsonian, Eclectic, and Physio-medical systems. This formula demonstrates how a small, core group of herbs can be manipulated to streamline the formula for a particular function.

The Expectorant Formulas

Use

- To facilitate coughing (produce a productive cough) by thinning the sputum.
- To promote the discharge of mucus from the respiratory passages.

Formulas

Dr. Christopher's Cough and Bronchitis Formula

Therapeutic Principle
Expectorant, resolve phlegm.

Constituents
- ¼ teaspoon Marshmallow (*Althea officinalis*)
- ½ teaspoon Coltsfoot (*Tussilago farfara*)
- ½ teaspoon Ground ivy (*Glechoma hederacea*)
- ½ teaspoon Licorice (*Glycyrrhiza glabra*)
- ½ teaspoon Elder flowers (*Sambucus canadensis*)

Form
Tea.

Dosage

Use one tablespoon or more as needed during coughing for irritation of the throat and use each hour afterwards. Prepare by infusing the herbs for 15 minutes in one pint of hot water, cover, and let stand until cool. Strain, sweeten with honey, bottle and keep in a cool place (Christopher, 1976).

Indication

Cough, cough with thin white sputum, salivation, chest distension, vertigo, sore throat, tickling in throat, irritation of throat. The pulse can be either slow and deep or slippery and wiry. The tongue usually appears with a white and slippery coating.

Application

Cough, bronchitis, sore and irritated throat, chronic bronchitis, common cold, influenza, emphysema.

Contraindication

Caution in pregnancy.

Herbs and Actions

The Tussilago acts as a diffusive expectorant, sedative, and demulcent. Althea acts as a soothing demulcent to support the action of the expectorants and pectorals. Sambucus acts as an alterative, mild diffusive, and relaxing diaphoretic (Priest, 1982). Licorice acts as a demulcent, expectorant, and synergist, harmonizing the different actions of the herbs in this formula. Ground Ivy acts as a pectoral, stimulant, tonic and diaphoretic.

Modification

With nausea or vomiting, add Ginger. With chronic pulmonary conditions, add Inula and Verbascum. With hayfever and asthma, add Verbascum, Inula, and Grindelia. With paroxysmal laryngeal cough, add Verbascum and Trifolium. With fever with dry, hot skin, add Achillea and Pulsatilla. With weakening night sweats, add Salvia (Priest, 1982).

Commentary

This is a good expectorant formula recorded my Dr. Christopher in ***School of Natural Healing***. The design of the formula is well thought through, and not just a variety of expectorant herbs thrown together in a hodgepodge. The expectorant herbs are protected and balanced by the addition of the soothing demulcent Althea. The Elder then acts as an alterative and diaphoretic, assisting in the body's cleansing and detoxifying from the illness. The Licorice acts also as a synergist and harmonizer, connecting the other herbs and potentizing their effect. The Ground Ivy also acts as a stomach tonic, assisting in the body's assimilation of these healing herbs.

Syrup of Horehound

Therapeutic Principle

Expectorant; clear phlegm.

Constituents

- 2 ounces Horehound (*Ballota nigra*)
- ½ ounce Licorice (*Glycyrrhiza glabra*)
- ½ ounce Polypodium of the Oak (*Polypodium vulgare*)
- ½ ounce Fennel (*Foeniculum vulgare*)
- ½ ounce Smallage root (*Apium graveolens*)
- 6 drams Maidenhair (*Adiantum pedatum*)
- 6 drams Origanum (*Origanum marjorana*)
- 6 drams Hyssop (*Hyssopus officinalis*)
- 6 drams Calaminth (*Calamintha acinos*)
- 6 drams Thyme (*Thymus vulgares*)
- 6 drams Savory (*Satureja hortensis*)
- 6 drams Scabious (*Knautia arvensis*)
- 6 drams Coltsfoot (*Tussilago farfara*)
- 3 drams Anise seeds (*Pimpinella anisum*)
- 3 drams Cotton seeds
- 2 ounces Raisins
- 10 Figs
- 8 pounds Hydromel
- 1 ounce Orris Florentine root (*Iris florentina*)

Form
Syrup

Dosage
Take one teaspoonful three times per day. To prepare, boil the herbs in eight pounds of hydromel, until half is boiled down, then boil the decoction into a syrup with two pounds each of honey and sugar. Perfume it with one ounce of the roots of Orris Florentine. Culpeper advised to take it with a Licorice stick.

Indication
Cough, white sputum, thick phlegm, averse to cold. Pulse tends to be slow and slippery. The tongue usually has a white and slippery coating.

Application
Cough, bronchitis, pneumonia, tuberculosis, common cold.

Contraindication
Contraindicated in pregnancy and acute kidney disease.

Herbs and Actions
These herbs act synergistically as an expectorant. Origanum acts as an expectorant, diaphoretic, and tonic. Hyssop acts as an expectorant, stimulant and tonic. Thyme acts as an expectorant and diaphoretic. Horehound acts as an expectorant, diaphoretic, stimulant, and tonic. Licorice acts as a demulcent and expectorant. Polypodium acts as a demulcent. Maidenhair acts as an expectorant and tonic. Fennel acts as an expectorant and stimulant. Smallage acts as a stimulant, diuretic, tonic, and nervine. Calaminth acts as an expectorant and diaphoretic. Coltsfoot acts as an expectorant, demulcent, and tonic. Savory acts as an expectorant. Scabious acts as an expectorant and diaphoretic. Anise acts as a pectoral and carminative. Orris acts as a diuretic and stomachic.

COMMENTARY

This is a formula from Culpeper, the great herbalist from the 17th century. In his ***Complete Herbal***, he records the properties and energetics of single herbs, formulas from Galen, Avicenna, and many other herbalists before and contemporary to him. He also has a commentary where he lists what the medical colleges say about a particular formula, followed by his commentary on the formula. For each formula, he gives recipes, or ways to prepare the particular formula, in very useful detail. Culpeper's comment to this formula is "It is appropriated to the breast and lungs, and is a fine cleanser to purge them from thick and putrified phlegm, it helps phthisicks and coughs, and diseases subject to old men, and cold natures. Take it with a Licorice stick (Culpeper, 1995)."

Friar's Balsam

THERAPEUTIC PRINCIPLE

Stimulating expectorant; antiseptic vulnerary; expectorant with moistening effect.

CONSTITUENTS

- Siam Benzoin resin (*Styrax tonkinensis*)
- Storax balsam (*Liquidambar orientalis*)
- Balsam of Tolu (*Toluifera balsamum*)
- Balsam of Peru (*Toluifera pareirae*)
- Aloe leaf latex (*Aloe barbadensis*)
- Myrrh tears (*Commiphora abyssinica*)
- Angelica root (*Angelica archangelica*) (Smith, 1997)

FORM

Balsam.

DOSAGE

Internally, take 30 drops three times per day in warm water. As an inhalant, mix two to three droppersful of the balsam into a pint of steaming water and breathe the vapors in deeply. As a topical, the cleaned wound should be covered with the balsam and gauze and changed daily (Smith, 1997).

INDICATION

Cough, phlegm, difficulty speaking, loss of voice, difficulty breathing, pain in chest, chapped skin and lips, cuts and abrasions, dry skin, itching skin, herpetic outbreaks. The pulse is usually superficial, while the tongue usually appears white with a thin coating.

APPLICATION

Cough, asthma, laryngitis, bronchitis, catarrh, cuts, abrasions, eczema, urticaria, chilblains, fissures, cracked nipples, chapped skin and lips, herpes simplex, indolent ulcers, bedsores, gingivitis (Smith, 1997).

CONTRAINDICATION

Avoid use with allergic skin conditions. If irritation does appear, discontinue use (Smith, 1997).

HERBS AND ACTIONS

Benzoin acts as a stimulating expectorant. Balsam of Tolu, Storax Balsam, and Balsam of Peru act as stimulating expectorants. Aloe Leaf acts as a purgative. Angelica acts as a stimulant, expectorant, stomachic, and tonic.

MODIFICATION

Jesuit's Drops are formed by using Benzoin, Balsam Tolu, Storax, Aloes and alcohol (Cook, 1869).

COMMENTARY

This six-hundred year old formula has been known by various names, including: Jesuit's Drops, Jerusalem Drops, Balsamic Tincture, Balsamum Traumaticum, Wound Balsam, St. Victor's Balsam, Commander's Balsam, Swedish Balsam, Persian Balsam, Wade's Balsam, Turlington's Balsam, and Wound Balsam (Smith, 1997).

Oxymel of Squills

Therapeutic Principle

Expectorant; eliminating wind and phlegm.

Constituents

- 5 drams Origanum (*Origanum marjorana*)
- 5 drams Hyssop (*Hyssopus officinalis*)
- 5 drams Thyme (*Thymus vulgares*)
- 5 drams Lovage (*Levisticum officinale*)
- 5 drams Cardamom (*Elettaria cardamomum*)
- 5 drams Stoechas (*Helichrysum stoechas*)
- 2 pounds Honey
- ½ pound Honey of Raisins
- 5 ounces Briony juice (*Bryonia dioica*)
- 1 ½ pound Vinegar of Squills (*Urginea scilla*)

Form

Syrup.

Dosage

Take one spoon three times per day. To prepare, boil the herbs in "three pounds of water to one, strain it and with two pounds of honey, honey of raisins half a pound, juice of Briony five ounces, Vinegar of Squills a pound and a half, boil it, and scum it according to art (Culpeper, 1995)."

Indication

Cough, dizziness, pain in the head, lung congestion, feeling of oppression and stuffiness in the chest, vertigo, profuse sputum. The pulse is usually soft and slippery. The tongue usually appears white with a greasy coating.

Application

Cough, bronchitis, vertigo, headache, neurotic vertigo, Meniere's disease.

Contraindication

Contraindicated for a patient with vertigo that is not caused by phlegm.

Herbs and Actions

Origanum acts as an expectorant, diaphoretic, and tonic. Hyssop acts as an expectorant, stimulant, and tonic. Thyme acts as an expectorant and diaphoretic. Lovage acts as an expectorant, diuretic, and stimulant. Cardamom acts as a stimulant and stomachic. Stoechas acts as an expectorant and deobstruent. Briony is a hydragogue and cathartic, useful in small doses for cough, bronchitis, pneumonia, influenza, pleurisy, and whooping cough, relieving pain and cough. Squills acts as an expectorant, stimulant, and diuretic.

Modification

By removing all other ingredients and just using the Vinegar of Squills, we have a nice and ancient remedy in itself. Culpeper, in his herbal, describes Galen's use of Vinegar of Squills:

"A little of this medicine being taken in the morning fasting, and walking half an hour after, preserves the body in health, to extreme old age, (as Sanius tried, who using no other medicine but this, lived in perfect health till one hundred and seventeen years of age), it makes the digestion good, a long wind, a clear voice, an acute sight, a good color, it suffers no offensive thing to remain in the body, neither wind, phlegm, choler, melancholy, dung, nor urine, but brings them forth; it brings forth filth though it lie in the bones, it takes away salt and sour belchings, though a man be never so licentious in diet, he shall feel no harm. It hath cured such as have the phthisic, that have been given over by all Physicians. It cures such as have the falling sickness, gouts, and diseases and swellings of the joints. It takes away the hardness of the liver and the spleen. We should never have done if we should reckon up the particular benefits of this medicine. Therefore we recommend it as a wholesome medicine for soundness of body, preservation of health, and vigour of mind. Thus Galen (Culpeper, 1995)."

Commentary

This formula shows up in both Culpeper's ***Complete Herbal*** and ***The Simmonite-Culpeper Herbal*** (1957). It was invented by Pythagoras, who lived in the sixth century before Christ (Grieves, 1931). Squill acts as a stimulant and expectorant. It was used by all of the ancient Greek physicians, and mentioned by Theophrastus in the third century before Christ. Dioscorides described how to make the vinegar of Squills, and similar compounds mixed with honey were administered by the Arabian physicians in the Middle Ages (Grieves, 1931). Culpeper (1995) comments on the formula by saying it "is good against the falling-sickness, Megrim, Head-ache, Vertigo, or swimming in the head, and if these be occasioned by the stomach as many times as they are, it helps the lungs obstructed by humour, and is good for women not well cleansed after labor, it opens the passage of the womb."

Expectorant Mixture

Therapeutic Principle

Expectorant; expel phlegm.

Constituents

- 2 drachms Compound Tincture of Camphor (*Cinnamomum camphora*)
- 2 drachms Oxymel of Squills
- 2 ounces Oxymel
- 2 ounces Mucilage of Acacia (*Acacia catechu*)

Form

Syrup.

Dosage

A tablespoonful when necessary.

Indication

Cough, wheezing, inflammation, fever, thirst, restlessness, edema, headache, fluid in the hypochondrium, pain in the chest and hypochrondria on coughing, shortness of breath, dizziness. The pulse can be tight or rapid, superficial or deep. The tongue usually has a thin white or yellow coating.

APPLICATION
Cough, common cold, pleurisy, influenza, edema, ascites.

CONTRAINDICATION
Contraindicated in pregnancy.

HERBS AND ACTIONS
Camphor acts as a respiratory circulation stimulant. Oxymel of Squills acts as an expectorant. Acacia acts as a respiratory demulcent.

MODIFICATION
The Oxymel of Squills can be used by itself without the pleurisy or edema.

COMMENTARY
This formula comes from ***The Simmonite-Culpeper Herbal*** (1957). It combines formulas from Culpeper's herbal to make a formula with a particular direction. As one glances through Culpeper's herbal, they can notice many formulas being combined to create a new formula with a different action, or a similar one with specific indications.

6

The Anti-tussive and Anti-asthmatic Formulas

Use

- To inhibit the excitatory state of the respiratory center and the cough reflex.
- To dilate the bronchi and the respiratory tract.

Formulas

Weiss' Cough Formula

Therapeutic Principle
Anti-tussive, with a moisturizing nature.

Constituents
- 1 part Mullein flowers (*Verbascum thapsus*)
- 1 part Coltsfoot (*Tussilago farfara*)
- 1 part Marshmallow root (*Althea officinalis*)
- 1 part Anise seed (*Pimpinella anisum*)

Form
Decoction.

Dosage
One cup three times per day.

Indication
Cough, dry cough with or without sputum, fever, headache, dry throat with thirst. The tongue tends to be dry and red with a thin white coating. The pulse is usually rapid and superficial.

Application
Cough, flu with a dry cough, upper respiratory tract infection, asthma.

Contraindication
Contraindicated with cough with chilliness and aversion to cold.

Herbs and Actions
Mullein acts as a demulcent and expectorant. Coltsfoot acts as an expectorant, demulcent, and tonic. Marshmallow acts as a demulcent and diuretic. Anise acts as a pectoral and carminative.

Modification
For cough with blood, add Agrimony. With hayfever and asthma, add Grindelia. With chronic pulmonary conditions, add Inula. With paroxysmal laryngeal cough, add Sambucus and Trifolium.

Commentary
This formula appeared with Rudolf Weiss, a great German herbalist of the Euro-science tradition. He is the author of ***Herbal Medicine***, a monumental work documenting the German herbal tradition of his time. Most of his influence came from Madaus.

Cough Drops

Therapeutic Principle
Anti-tussive.

Constituents
- 4 ounces Lobelia (*Lobelia inflata*)
- 2 ounces Horehound (*Marrubium vulgare*)
- 2 ounces Comfrey (*Symphytum officinale*)
- 2 ounces Elecampane (*Inula helenium*)
- 4 ounces Boneset (*Eupatorium perfoliatum*)

Form
Decoction.

Dosage
Two to three teaspoonfuls once an hour. To prepare, boil the herbs in three quarts of water down to three pints. Strain and add two pounds of sugar and one pint of gin.

Indication
Cough, dry cough, fever, headache, body aches. The pulse is usually weak, thready, or rapid. The tongue is usually red and dry with a thin white coating.

Application
Cough, influenza with cough, asthma, upper respiratory tract infection, croup, pertussis, tuberculosis.

Contraindication
Contraindicated in pregnancy.

HERBS AND ACTIONS
Inula and Marrubium act as tonic expectorants. Symphytum acts as a soothing demulcent. Eupatorium acts a stimulating, tonic, and anti-spasmodic diaphoretic. Lobelia acts as a general systemic relaxant with diffusive stimulation (Priest, 1982).

MODIFICATION
With hemoptysis, add Calendula. With night sweats and aching bones, add Achillea for the first stage and Pulsatilla during the third stage. With chest soreness and pulmonary inflammation, add Asclepias and Inula. With pertussis, add Trifolium. With chronic cough in the elderly, add Sticta. With bronchitis and catarrh, add Prunus (Priest, 1982).

COMMENTARY
This formula is from Samuel Thomson, the founder of the Thomsonian herbal system of the early 19th century. He influenced millions of people with his herbals and home health books. Many medical doctors practiced Thomsonian herbalism, and then broke off into the professional branch known as the Physio-Medicalists.

Compounded Stillingia Liniment

THERAPEUTIC PRINCIPLE
Anti-tussive.

CONSTITUENTS
- 4 parts Queens root (*Stillingia sylvatica*)
- 1 part Indian tobacco (*Lobelia inflata*)
- 2 parts White tea tree (*Meleleuca leucodendron*) oil
- 6 parts alcohol
- 6 parts vegetable glycerin

FORM
Tincture

DOSAGE
Take 15-30 drops three times per day.

Indication
Cough, dry cough with little or no sputum, dry throat and nostrils. The pulse is usually weak or thready. The tongue usually appears red and dry, maybe with a thin white coating.

Application
Cough, bronchial asthma, upper respiratory tract infection, croup, pertussis, pleurisy.

Contraindication
Contraindicated in pregnancy.

Herbs and Actions
Melaleuca acts as an expectorant. Lobelia is a general systemic relaxant with diffusive stimulation, indicated in bronchitis, pleurisy, pertussis, bronchial asthma, and spasmodic and membranous croup. Stillingia is an alterative and influences secretory functions.

Modification
For chronic bronchitis or laryngitis, add oil of Anise or Caraway (Grieves, 1931). By removing the Lobelia and Melaleuca, and adding Turkey Corn, Iris, Elder flowers, Pipsissewa, Coriander, and Prickly Ash, we have compound syrup of Stillingia, a powerful alterative (Cook, 1869).

Commentary
This is an all-purpose respiratory formula with strong alterative qualities, remarkably effective for croup, bronchitis, and other acute upper respiratory conditions. It is also useful externally for musculoskeletal complaints (Boyle, 1993).

Spezies Grippales Compositum

Therapeutic Principle
Anti-tussive.

Constituents
- Mullein (*Verbascum thapsus*)
- Horehound (*Marrubium vulgare*)
- Fennel (*Foeniculum vulgare*)
- Dill (*Peucedanum graveolens*)

Form
Decoction.

Dosage
One cup three times per day.

Indication
Cough, fever, hiccough with dyspnea, dry throat. The pulse can be rapid or thready, sometimes superficial. The tongue usually has a thin white coating.

Application
Cough, influenza with cough, upper respiratory tract infection.

Contraindication
None known.

Herbs and Actions
Horehound acts as a gently diffusive tonic expectorant. Mullein acts as a demulcent, alterative, and diuretic. Fennel acts as a carminative and aromatic, opening the orifices of the head. It also has an effect upon chronic coughs (Grieves, 1931). Dill also acts as an aromatic and carminative, but also is a stimulant and effective for hiccoughs.

Modification

With hayfever or asthma, add Grindelia. With paroxysmal cough, add Trifolium or Sambucus. With catarrh or bronchitis, add Prunus or Inula.

Commentary

This 11th century formula from Hildegard von Bingen is very effective for coughs. Hildegard lived in a monastery in Germany and, through a series of visions inspired by God, developed a type of medicine called Veriditas, or Green Medicine, in which herbs, minerals, and diet are employed, along with their energetic properties (Strehlow, 1988).

Cough Powder

Therapeutic Principle

Anti-tussive with a warming nature.

Constituents

- ¼ ounce Cayenne (*Capsicum frutescens*)
- 1 ounce Lobelia (*Lobelia inflata*)
- 2 ounce Slippery Elm (*Ulmus fulva*)
- 1 ounce Skunk Cabbage (*Symplocarpus foetida*)
- 1 ounce Wake Robin (*Trillium pendulum*)
- 1 ounce Valerian (*Valeriana officinalis*)
- 1 ounce Prickly Ash (*Xanthoxylum americanum*)

Form

Powder

Dosage

Half a teaspoonful in hot water, once every two or three hours.

Indication

Cough, asthma, intolerance of cold, pale face, low energy, voice low and weak. The pulse is usually weak and feeble. The tongue can be pale with a thin white coating.

Application
Cough, tuberculosis, asthma, croup, laryngitis.

Contraindication
Contraindicated in pregnancy.

Herbs and Actions
Lobelia acts as a general systemic relaxant, while Cayenne and Prickly Ash act as general stimulants. Wake Robin acts as an astringent tonic. Lobelia, Skunk Cabbage, and Cayenne all act as expectorants. Slippery Elm is a demulcent, providing protection against the expectorants and stimulants. Valerian acts as a nervine, sedative, and anti-spasmodic.

Modification
With swollen glands, add Phytolacca. With insomnia, add Humulus.

Commentary
This Thomsonian Formula appeared in Benjamin Colby's (1846) book, ***A Guide to Health***. It is made up of a variety of herbs that are geared towards tonifying the lung while being an anti-tussive.

Asthma Formula

Therapeutic Principle
Anti-tussive and anti-asthmatic.

Constituents
- ½ ounce Elecampane root (*Inula helenium*)
- ½ ounce Comfrey root (*Symphytum officinale*)
- ½ ounce Horehound (*Marrubium vulgare*)
- ½ ounce Black Cohosh (*Cimicifuga racemosa*)
- ½ ounce Spikenard (*Aralia racemosa*)
- ½ ounce Skunk Cabbage (*Symplocarpus foetida*)

Form
Decoction.

Dosage

One cupful every three to four hours. To prepare, pour three pints of boiling water over the herbs and steep for one hour. Strain and sweeten with honey.

Indication

Cough, asthma, fever, dry throat, thirsty. The pulse tends to be superficial, rapid, and slippery. The tongue usually has a thin white or yellow coating.

Application

Asthma, bronchitis, pneumonia, upper respiratory tract infection.

Contraindication

Contraindicated in pregnancy and for a patient with asthma with a cold nature.

Herbs and Actions

Inula acts as an expectorant, antiasthmatic, diaphoretic and tonic. Symphytum is a soothing demulcent, allaying irritation. Marrubium is an expectorant and pectoral, combining well with Inula for colds, bronchitis, and catarrh. Cimicifuga acts as an anti -spasmodic, alterative, and expectorant. Aralia is a diaphoretic and stimulant expectorant.

Modification

For pertussis or chorea, add Cypripedium or Caulophyllum. For bronchitis, remove the Cimicifuga and Symplocarpus, and add Prunus.

Commentary

This formula appeared in Dr. Christopher's herbal. Dr. Christopher was an influential herbalist of the latter part of the twentieth century. His herbals record numerous formulas from his teachers and that he formulated. He was well-versed in Thomsonian Herbalism and Physio-Medical Herbalism, having studied at Dominion Herbal College in Canada.

Katuah Asthma Formula

Therapeutic Principle
Anti-asthmatic.

Constituents
- Indian Turnip (*Arisaema triphyllum*)
- Hickory bark (*Carya tomentosa*)
- Maidenhair (*Adiantum pedatum*)
- Honey

Form
Decoction.

Dosage
One tablespoon three to four times per day. To prepare, boil the hickory bark in one quart of water for 15 minutes. Add the other herbs, strain, and add honey.

Indication
Cough, asthma, fever, with or without perspiration, thirsty, dry throat. The pulse is usually superficial, rapid, and slippery. The tongue tends to have a thin white or yellow coat.

Application
Asthma, cough, pneumonia, chronic bronchitis, upper respiratory tract infection.

Contraindication
Contraindicated in pregnancy. Do not use the Arisaema in the fresh state, it is a violent irritant to the mucus membranes.

Herbs and Actions

Arisaema acts as an expectorant, stimulant, and diaphoretic. It is a stimulant to the lungs, and the honey is given due to Arisaema's acrimony. The Maidenhair acts as an expectorant, refrigerant, and tonic. The Hickory acts as a diaphoretic and stomach tonic, allowing the Arisaema to be digested.

Modification

With high temperature, asthma, and cough, add Goldenseal. With dyspnea, add Mullein.

Commentary

This is a Cherokee formula, hence the name Katuah, meaning the Southern Appalachian bioregion. It also shows up in Thomas Deschauer's ***Complete Course in Herbalism***. The Cherokee practiced an advanced form of herbal medicine.

Kuts-Cheraux Asthma Formula

Therapeutic Principle

Anti-asthmatic.

Constituents

- Grindelia (*Grindelia robusta*)
- Flowering Spurge (*Euphorbia corollata*)
- Elecampane (*Inula helenium*)

Form

Tincture.

Dosage

Thirty Drops three times per day.

Indications

Wheezing, harsh, dry and unproductive cough, sense of constriction in the chest.

APPLICATION

Asthma, allergies, bronchial edema, upper respiratory tract infection.

HERBS AND ACTIONS

Grindelia guides the other herbs to the upper respiratory tract and acts as an expectorant and respiratory stimulant. Flowering Spurge acts as an expectorant and diaphoretic. Elecampane acts as an expectorant and anti-tussive.

MODIFICATIONS

Remove Flowering Spurge and add Echinacea and Licorice for upper respiratory tract infections.

COMMENTARY

This formula is recorded in ***Naturae Medicina*** by Dr. Kuts-Cheraux. The book is a Materia Medica developed by a committee of the American Association of Naturopathic Physicians and Surgeons in 1953. It also includes information donated by Dr. H. Riley Spitler, the author of ***Standardized Naturopathy***.

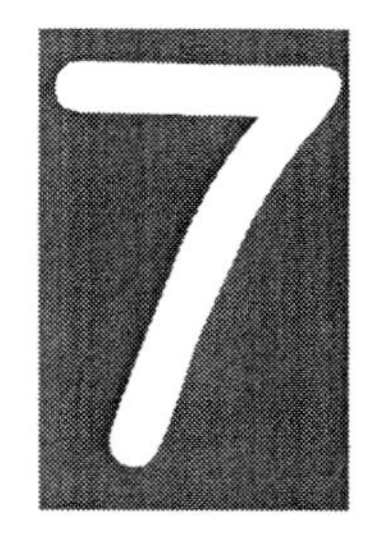

The Warming Formulas

Use

- To generally warm the body and increase metabolism.
- To aid decreased body temperature, cold extremities, very weak pulse, diarrhea, vomiting.

Formulas

Colby's Composition Powder

Therapeutic Principle
Stimulant; warm the stomach formula; tonic.

Constituents
- 2 pounds Bayberry (*Myrica cerifera*)
- 1 pound Ginger (*Zingiber officinale*)
- 2 ounces Cayenne (*Capsicum minimum*)
- 2 ounces Cinnamon (*Cinnamomum zeylanicum*)
- 2 ounces Prickly Ash (*Xanthoxylum americanum*)

Form
Powder.

Dosage
Take one teaspoon in two-thirds of a cup of hot water, sweetened (Colby, 1846).

Indication
Abdominal pain, fullness in the epigastric region, loss of appetite, headache, the first stages of colds, obstructions caused by cold, chilliness, acid regurgitation. The pulse tends to be slow and weak. The tongue is usually pale with a white and maybe slippery coat.

Application
Acute and chronic gastritis, headache, common cold, anemia, dysentery, abscesses, poor circulation, blood poisoning.

Contraindication
Contraindicated for diseases of a hot nature.

Herbs and Actions
The Bayberry acts as an alterative, stimulant, and tonic astringent. The Cayenne and Ginger act as general stimulants. The Prickly Ash is a stimulant with a warm and pungent nature. The Cayenne, Ginger, Cinnamon, and Prickly Ash are all warming agents (Colby, 1846).

Modification
By removing the Prickly Ash and Cinnamon, and replacing with Pinus and Cloves, one has Dr. Nowell's Composition Powder. By increasing the amounts of Bayberry and Ginger, it can be directed towards elder patients and is good for lumbar pain and urinary tract infections.

Commentary
This formula is from Dr. Colby, who studied under Dr. Samuel Thomson, the founder of the Thomsonian herbal system in the early 19th century. Composition Powder has been used as the base of many formulas since Dr. Thomson developed it. This is one modification that has a more warming nature.

Composition or Vegetable Powder

Therapeutic Principle
Stimulant; warm the stomach formula.

Constituents
- 2 pounds Bayberry root bark (*Myrica cerifera*)
- 1 pound Hemlock spruce inner bark (*Tsuga canadensis*)
- 1 pound Ginger (*Zingiber officinale*)
- 2 ounces Cayenne (*Capsicum minimum*)
- 2 ounces Cloves (*Syzygium aromaticum*)

Form
Powder.

Dosage
Take one teaspoon in ½ a cup of boiling water. Drink as soon as cool.

Indication
Abdominal pain, abdominal distension, fullness in the epigastric region, headache, first stages of a cold, cold extremities, loss of appetite, diarrhea. The pulse is slow and weak. The tongue usually appears light with a white coat.

Application
Acute and chronic gastritis, common cold, dysentery, diarrhea, chronic colitis.

Contraindication
Contraindicated in conditions of a hot nature.

Herbs and Actions
The herbs act together as a warming stimulant, tonic, and astringent. Bayberry acts as an alterative, stimulant, and tonic astringent. The Cayenne and Ginger are warming, and act as general stimulants. The Hemlock acts as an astringent and diuretic. The Cloves act as an aromatic and stimulant.

MODIFICATION

Remove the Pinus for more of a diaphoretic action. Remove the Cloves and Cayenne for diarrhea, dysentery, hemorrhoids, and colitis (Christopher, 1976).

COMMENTARY

This formula is from Dr. Samuel Thomson, the founder of Thomsonian herbalism and probably the most influential American herbalist, having influenced and shaped whole schools of thought over the last 150 years. He developed a "course of medicine" in eight formulas:

Formula One	The Emetic (Lobelia)
Formula Two	Cayenne Pepper
Formula Three	The Canker Remedy (Bayberry, White Pond Lily, and Hemlock Bark)
Formula Four	Bitters (Balmony, Bayberry and Poplar Bark)
Formula Five	Syrup (Poplar Bark, Bayberry, Ground Cherry Stones)
Formula Six	Special Drops (Myrrh, Cayenne, Brandy)
Formula Seven	Composition Powder
Formula Eight	Nerve Powder (Lady's Slipper)

He developed his own theory of disease, feeling that disease was started by cold and a decrease in vital fluids, which caused an obstruction or canker, leading to disease, putrefaction, or death. Disease could be reversed by restoring the vital energy, which was done by restoring the body's vital heat and using emetics. Dr. Thomson used not only herbalism, but also enemas, steam baths, hydrotherapy, and emesis.

The Digestive Formulas

Use

- As digestive formulas.
- To increase the digestion of fat, protein, and carbohydrates.
- To enhance the appetite.
- To increase the secretion of gastric acid.
- To increase digestion and evacuation.

Formulas

Dr. Carroll's "50" Capsules

THERAPEUTIC PRINCIPLE

To promote the digestive function of the stomach and remove stagnated food.

CONSTITUENTS

- 2 parts Gentian (*Gentiana lutea*)
- 1 part Skullcap (*Scutellaria lateriflora*)

FORM

Capsule.

Dosage
One "00" Capsule in warm water.

Indication
Poor digestion related to stress, decreased appetite, flatulence. For food stagnation with symptoms of belching, fullness and distension in the gastric region, acid regurgitation, loss of appetite, constipation or diarrhea. The tongue tends to have a yellow and greasy coating and the pulse tends to be slippery. Nerve rings can be present in the iris.

Application
Indigestion, flatulence, abdominal pain, gastrointestinal flu, nervous stomach, diarrhea, loss of appetite.

Contraindication
Contraindicated for gastric and abdominal distension due to deficiency or malnutrition.

Herbs and actions
The Gentian improves the appetite and digestion by increasing HCl production in the stomach. The Skullcap calms the nerves and beneficially influences the gastrointestinal tract, especially the stomach, via the nervous system (Boyle, 1988).

Modification
With more insomnia and less digestive stress, remove the Gentian and add one part Valerian; this produces Dr. Carroll's "Nervine Capsules." With gastric oppression and fullness, add orange peel. With bad breath, add Goldenseal or Oregon Grape. With constipation add one part Cape Aloes.

Commentary
This is a classic small formula handed down to the naturopathic community from Dr. O.G. Carroll. Dr. Harold Dick preserved it and passed it on to a couple of generations of Naturopaths. All of Dr. Carroll's formulas have been used classically with constitutional hydrotherapy, a method developed by Dr. Carroll and taught at all of the Naturopathic medical schools.

Gentian and Ginger Combination

Therapeutic Principle

To promote the digestive function of the stomach and remove stagnated food.

Constituents

- Gentian (*Gentiana lutea*)
- Ginger (*Zingiber officinalis*)

Form

Tincture or capsule.

Dosage

Thirty drops or two capsules before meals.

Indication

Poor digestion, decreased appetite, flatulence, bloating, acid regurgitation, constipation, diarrhea, allergies. The tongue tends to have a yellow coating and the pulse tends to be slippery.

Application

Indigestion, flatulence, abdominal pain, gastrointestinal flu, diarrhea, loss of appetite, hypochlorhydria.

Contraindication

Contraindicated for gastric and abdominal distension due to deficiency or malnutrition.

Herbs and Actions

The Gentian improves the appetite and digestion by increasing HCl production in the stomach. Ginger improves digestion and warms the stomach.

Modification

With nervousness, remove the Ginger and add Skullcap.

Commentary

This classic small formula may be the most prescribed formula. It has been given to many patients simply to improve digestion, assimilation, and nutrition, which are cornerstones to health in Naturopathy.

Spiced Bitters

Therapeutic Principle

Digestive.

Constituents

- 2 pounds Poplar bark (*Populus tremuloides*)
- 8 ounces Goldenseal (*Hydrastis canadensis*)
- 12 ounces Prickly Ash bark (*Xanthoxylum americana*)
- 8 ounces Ginger (*Zingiber officinale*)
- 8 ounces Cloves (*Syzygium aromatica*)
- 4 ounces Cinnamon (*Cinnamomum zeylanicum*)
- 8 ounces Balmony (*Chelone glabra*)
- 6 ounces Cayenne (*Capsicum minimum*)
- 5 pounds Sugar

Form

Powder.

Dosage

Take one teaspoonful of the powder in half a cup of hot water three times per day, before meals. To prepare, pulverize the herbs, sift and mix (Colby, 1846).

Indication

Indigestion, loss of appetite, malaise, weakness, fullness and distension in the gastric region, belching, acid regurgitation, constipation or diarrhea. The pulse tends to be slippery. The tongue usually appears yellow with a greasy coating.

APPLICATION

Loss of appetite, indigestion, jaundice, nausea, bloating, diarrhea, abdominal pain, gastrointestinal flu.

CONTRAINDICATION

Fever, tight sensation of the lungs, abdominal distension due to malnutrition and deficiency.

HERBS AND ACTIONS

The herbs as a whole act as a tonic compound. They are warming, stimulating, astringing, and tonifying. The Poplar acts as a stomachic and tonic (Lust, 1974). The Balmony acts as a tonic with specific action on the liver and intestinal areas (Christopher, 1976).

MODIFICATION

With bad breath, add Berberis. With flu symptoms, add Boneset.

COMMENTARY

This formula comes from the Thomsonian system of herbalism. It is considered "an excellent tonic compound, useful in all cases of indigestion, loss of appetite, jaundice, general debility, and all other cases where the system is in a weak, relaxed state (Colby, 1846)."

The Tonifying Formulas

Use

- To tonify the vital force.
- To tonify blood.
- To increase metabolism.
- To act on the immune system.
- To increase adaptability of the body.
- To tonify the endocrine and nervous systems.
- To reduce stress and fatigue, increase memory.

Formulas

Breakfast Tea

THERAPEUTIC PRINCIPLE
Tonify the body's vital energy.

CONSTITUENTS
- 50 g Rose hips (*Rosa spp.*)
- 20 g Strawberry leaves (*Fragaria vesca*)
- 20 g Linden blossoms (*Tilia europaea or americana*)
- 10 g Thyme (*Thymus vulgaris*)

Form
Tea.

Dosage
Mix together, pour one cup boiling water over one to two teaspoons of herbs, let steep for three to five minutes, strain, stir in honey to taste, drink one cup hot in the morning.

Indication
A general prophylactic for healthy people.

Application
Tonify the general systems of the body, prophylaxis.

Contraindication
Must be modified for illness.

Herbs and Actions
The Strawberry Leaves and Thyme promote digestion. The Thyme also inhibits fermentation and disinfects the throat. The Rose Hips stimulate the kidneys and cleanse the blood. The Linden Blossoms elevate the skin's function.

Modification
Add Craetagus as a heart and circulatory system tonic. Add Milk Thistle as a liver tonic.

Commentary
This first appears with Erich Rauch, MD, a German practitioner of naturopathic medicine. It is a general tonic to be used in states of well-being without illness. Dr. Rauch also employed nature cure methods with his treatments, such as enemas, baths, and other hydrotherapeutic techniques.

Glyconda (Neutralizing Cordial)

THERAPEUTIC PRINCIPLE
Tonify the body's vital energy, laxative, antacid, alterative.

CONSTITUENTS
- 2 parts Indian rhubarb (*Rheum pelatum*)
- 2 parts Potassium bicarbonate
- 1 part Goldenseal (*Hydrastis canadensis*)
- 1 part Cinnamon (*Cinnamomum cassia*)
- 1/32 part Peppermint (*Mentha piperita*) oil in a glycerin, alcohol, and water base (Boyle, 1993)

FORM
Tincture.

DOSAGE
As a soothing gastrointestinal corrective, take 30-60 drops every half hour to two hours in four ounces of water, according to urgency of symptoms. As a laxative, use one tablespoonful in a cup of water. For diarrhea, dosages should not exceed 80 drops (Smith).

INDICATION
Loose stool, belching, gas, nausea, constipation, bloating, abdominal pain, distension, undigested food in stool, acid regurgitation, loss of taste and appetite, malaise. The pulse tends to be either moderate or slippery, and the tongue usually has a white, greasy coating.

APPLICATION
Diarrhea, constipation, muco-enteritis, vomiting, nausea, food stagnation, sour stomach, dysentery, gastritis.

CONTRAINDICATION
Contraindicated for abdominal and gastric bloating due to deficiency and malnutrition.

HERBS AND ACTIONS
The herbs in this formula act synergistically as a laxative, alterative, antacid, and tonic.

MODIFICATION
For indigestion, add Orange Peel and Licorice. For indigestion and prefers heat, add Orange Peel and Ginger. For indigestion following consumption of meat, add Crataegus. For indigestion with bad breath, add Oregon Grape or Goldenseal.

COMMENTARY
This formula from the Eclectic school was the Tums of the nineteenth century (Boyle, 1993). It acts as a laxative, antacid, and tonic. It has alterative effects on the gastrointestinal tract and is useful for both constipation and diarrhea. Its pleasant taste has made it a popular vehicle for administering bad tasting preparations to children. This is a modification of Locke's Neutralizing Cordial, which contained Rhubarb, Peppermint, Potassium Bicarbonate, Essence of Peppermint, sugar, and alcohol (Felter, 1922).

Cherokee Blood Tonic

THERAPEUTIC PRINCIPLE
Tonify the blood.

CONSTITUENTS
- Yellowroot (*Xanthorhiza simplicissima*)
- Red Alder (*Alnus serrulata*)
- Rattlesnake Plantain (*Goodyera pubescens*)
- Wild Ginger (*Asarum canadense*)
- Wild Cherry (*Prunus virginica*)

FORM
Decoction.

DOSAGE
Take one cup three times per day.

INDICATION
Pale face, lips and fingernails, dizziness, anemia, insomnia, lack of appetite, irregular menstruation, decreased flow of blood, abdominal pain, amenorrhea.

APPLICATION
Anemia, aplastic anemia, chronic bleeding, menorrhagia, uterine bleeding, gastric and duodenal ulcer, functional uterine bleeding, irregular menstruation.

CONTRAINDICATION
Contraindicated in pregnancy.

HERBS AND ACTIONS
The Red Alder and Cherry act as blood tonifiers. The Yellowroot acts as an astringent and tonic. The Wild Ginger is a stimulant with specific therapeutic actions as a female regulator. Rattlesnake Plantain improves the appetite and is tonic to the kidneys (Chiltoskey, 1975).

MODIFICATION
Add Sassafras to enhance the effect of blood tonification.

COMMENTARY
This is a Cherokee formula from the Eastern Band. It was used as a good blood tonic and for many menstrual problems. The Doctrine of Signatures can be seen at work with the use of the Red Alder and Wild Cherry as blood tonics.

Dr. Carroll's Blood Tonic

Therapeutic Principle
Tonify the blood.

Constituents
- 1 cup Pipsissewa (dry cut) (*Chimaphila umbellata*)
- 1 cup Echinacea (*Echinacea spp.*)
- ½ cup Gentian (*Gentiana lutea*)
- ½ cup Podophyllum (*Podophyllum peltatum*)

Form
Decoction.

Dosage
Take one tablespoon three times per day. To prepare, add the herbs to eleven pints of water and boil for five to ten minutes. Strain, add oil of wintergreen to taste, bottle, and keep refrigerated (Boyle, 1988).

Indication
Pale face, dizziness, shortness of breath, general fatigue, palpitation, loss of appetite. The pulse tends to be thready and weak. The tongue usually appears light with a thin white coating.

Application
Chronic diseases, anemia, irregular menstruation, uterine bleeding, liver congestion.

Contraindication
Contraindicated in pregnancy.

Herbs and Actions

Echinacea acts as an alterative, blood tonic, blood purifier, and immune enhancer. Pipsissewa acts as a tonic, alterative, astringent and diuretic. It is a specific tonic to the cardiovascular system. Gentian acts as an emmenagogue, bitter tonic, and strengthens the human system. It is combined with the Mayapple to prevent the debilitating effects of its purgative and cathartic actions. Mayapple acts as a liver stimulant, relieving congested states (Grieves, 1931).

Modification

With irregular menstruation and abdominal pain during menstruation, leukorrhea, back pain, fatigue, decreased appetite, add Mother's wort. For coldness of the body, add Cinnamon.

Commentary

This formula is from Dr. O.G. Carroll, a great naturopath from the early part of this century. He had a profound effect upon modern naturopathy, especially as preserved in the teachings of Dr. Harold Dick of Spokane.

Spiced Bitters

Therapeutic Principle

Tonify the stomach and vital energy.

Constituents

- Poplar bark (*Populus tremuloides*)
- Goldenseal (*Hydrastis canadensis*)
- Prickly Ash bark (*Xanthoxylum americana*)
- Ginger (*Zingiber officinale*)
- Cloves (*Syzygium aromaticum*)
- Cinnamon (*Cinnamomum zeylanica*)
- Balmony (*Chelone glabra*)
- Cayenne (*Capsicum minimum*)

Form

Powder.

Dosage

Take one teaspoon in half a cup of hot water three times daily, before eating.

Indication

Loss of appetite, diarrhea, pale face, muscle weakness, indigestion, abdominal distension, borborygmus. The pulse tends to be weak and the tongue usually has a light color with a thin coating.

Application

Chronic gastritis, indigestion, general debility, loss of appetite.

Contraindication

Contraindicated in pregnancy.

Herbs and Actions

The herbs act together as a tonic and stomachic, with stimulant and astringing properties. Poplar acts as a stomachic and tonic. Goldenseal acts as a tonic and bitter. Prickly Ash acts as an alterative and stimulant. Ginger acts as an appetizer, adjuvant, carminative, sialagogue, and stimulant. Cloves are warming, aromatic, and spicy, acting as a digestive. Cinnamon is warming, stimulating, and promotes assimilation. Balmony acts as an aperient, stimulant, and tonic. Cayenne functions as an appetizer, digestive, sialagogue, stimulant, and tonic.

Modifications

With weakness, add Orange peel.

Commentary

This is a Thomsonian formula that has been used effectively for over 150 years. It is an example of the combination of local and exotic plants that was occurring in the early 19th century in the Americas, where Samuel Thomson was combining American Indian herbal medicine with European herbal medicine.

Dr. Coffin's Stomach Bitters

THERAPEUTIC PRINCIPLE
Tonify the stomach.

CONSTITUENTS
- 4 ounces Bayberry bark (*Myrica cerifera*)
- 4 ounces Balmony, powder (*Chelone glabra*)
- 2 ounces Poplar bark, powder (*Populus tremuloides*)
- 2 ounces Ginger (*Zingiber officinale*)
- ¼ ounce Cayenne (*Capsicum minimum*)
- ¼ ounce Cloves (*Syzygium aromatica*)

FORM
Powder.

DOSAGE
Take one cupful warm three times daily (Christopher, 1976). Use one teaspoon of the compound in one cupful of hot water, cover and steep a few minutes, sweeten with honey to taste.

INDICATION
Loss of appetite, general fatigue, flatulence, chronic disease. The pulse is usually weak, and the tongue appears light with a thin coating.

APPLICATION
Loss of appetite, flatulence, abdominal bloating and pain, chronic gastritis, liver congestion, diarrhea.

CONTRAINDICATION
Contraindicated in pregnancy.

Herbs and Actions
The herbs act synergistically as a stomach tonic, with stimulant and astringent properties (Colby, 1846). Bayberry acts as a tonic, stimulant, and astringent. Balmony acts as an aperient, stimulant, and tonic. Poplar acts as a stomachic and tonic. Ginger acts as an appetizer, adjuvant, carminative, sialagogue, and stimulant. Cayenne acts as an appetizer, digestive, sialagogue, stimulant, and tonic. Cloves are warming, aromatic, and spicy, acting as a digestive.

Modification
For bad breath, add Goldenseal and Berberis. For weakness, add Orange peel. Remove Ginger, Cayenne, and Cloves to form Thomson's Bitters.

Commentary
This formula's roots come from Samuel Thomson, the founder of Thomsonian herbalism in the early 19th century. Dr. Coffin modified it by adding Ginger, Cayenne, and Cloves. Dr. Coffin studied under Samuel Thomson, and later went to England, spreading Thomsonian Medical Herbalism.

Kidney Tonic

Therapeutic Principle
Tonify the kidney.

Constituents
- 1 ounce Uva Ursi (*Arctostaphylos uva-ursi*)
- 1 ounce Goldenrod (*Solidago odora*)
- ½ ounce Prince's Pine (*Chimaphila umbellata*)
- ½ ounce Licorice root (*Glycyrrhiza glabra*)
- 1 ounce Buchu (*Barosma betulina*)
- 1 teaspoon Cayenne (*Capsicum minimum*)

Form
Decoction.

Dosage

One cup warm three times per day and before bed. To prepare, simmer the first four herbs slowly in three pints of water, then pour hot over the Buchu and Cayenne and steep until cool, then strain (Christopher, 1976).

Indication

Low back pain, dizziness, dry mouth, tinnitis, night perspiration. The pulse is usually thready and rapid. The tongue usually appears red and dry with a thin coating.

Application

Lumbago, chronic urinary tract infection, tinnitis, kidney infections.

Contraindication

Contraindicated with hyperactive states.

Herbs and Actions

The herbs act synergistically to tonify the kidneys and urinary tract. They have diuretic, warming, and stimulating properties. Uva Ursi acts as a kidney tonic. Goldenrod acts as an aromatic relaxant and diuretic. Prince's Pine acts as a kidney tonic and alterative. Licorice acts as a demulcent and relaxant, also calming Cayenne. Buchu acts as a tonic and nervine to the urinary tract. Cayenne acts as a stimulant and is indicated in chronic conditions of the kidneys.

Modification

With constipation, add ¼ ounce Cascara Bark. With severe weakness, add Cinnamon.

Commentary

This formula appears in Dr. Christopher's book (1976). It is based upon Thomsonian and Physio-Medical herbalism, using herbs in a classical fashion. Tonification of the kidney is extremely important, considering it is such a vital organ. Sweet Goldenrod (an odor similar to Anise) must be used, not just any Goldenrod species (Moore, 1988).

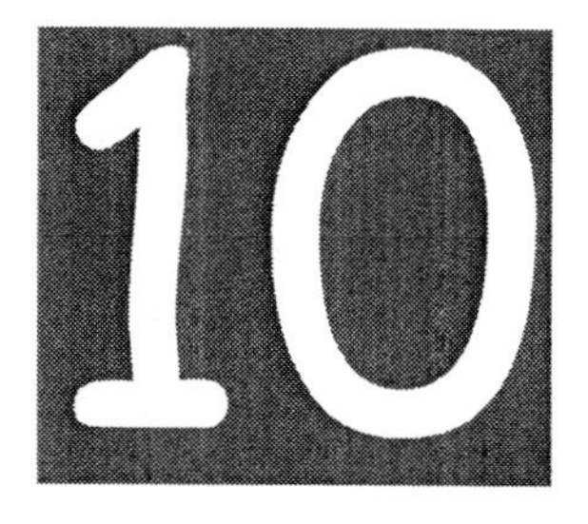

The Carminative Formulas

Use

- For local pain, distension, or oppression.
- To regulate action of the digestive tract.
- To relax the smooth muscles.
- As a cholagogue, increasing the secretion of bile.

Formulas

Carminative Drops

THERAPEUTIC PRINCIPLE
Carminative and digestive.

CONSTITUENTS
- 4 ounces Angelica (*Angelica archangelica*)
- 2 ounces Dioscorea (*Dioscorea villosa*)
- 1 ounce Mothersworth (*Leonurus cardiaca*)
- 1 ounce Coriander (*Coriandrum sativum*)
- 1 ounce Anise seeds (*Pimpinella anisum*)
- 1 ounce Dill seeds (*Peucadanum graveolens*)

Form

Compound tincture. Crush the herbs, macerate in forty ounces of 30% alcohol for ten days. Strain and add two pounds of sugar to the clear liquid.

Dosage

One-half to one teaspoon per hour.

Indication

Flatulence, colic, abdominal pain without inflammation, epigastric fullness and oppression, indigestion, belching, abdominal distension, acid regurgitation. The pulse tends to be wiry and taut. The tongue is usually greasy or slippery, with a thin coating.

Application

Indigestion, gastric or duodenal ulcer, chronic gastritis, cholecystitis, gastrointestinal neurosis, nausea.

Contraindication

Contraindicated for a person with food stagnation due to weakness.

Herbs and Actions

Angelica is aromatic and pungent, stimulating and relaxing to the stomach, relieving flatulence and wind colic. Dioscorea combines with Angelica, and it acts as an anti-spasmodic, assisting in the relief of flatus. Leonurus acts as a tonic and stimulant upon the stomach, promoting appetite and digestion. The three seeds act as carminatives.

Modification

For pain in the hypochondrium and a yellow tongue coating, add Corydalis. For flatulent dyspepsia, add Alpinia. With sour stomach and diarrhea, add equal parts of Neutralizing Cordial.

COMMENTARY

This formula appeared with William Cook, the great physician from the Physio-Medicalist school of therapeutic herbalism. The formula appeared in his book, ***The Physio-Medical Dispensatory*** (Cook, 1869). He felt that "This is an agreeable and a most reliable carminative preparation for all forms of flatulence, colic, and abdominal pains not connected with inflammation (Cook, 1869)."

Children's Herb Tea

THERAPEUTIC PRINCIPLE

Carminative.

CONSTITUENTS

- Fennel seed (*Foeniculum vulgare*)
- Chamomile (*Anthemis nobilis*)
- Sweet Weed (*Polygonum hydropiper*)
- Licorice (*Glycyrrhiza glabra*)

FORM

Decoction.

DOSAGE

One teaspoon three times per day.

INDICATION

Gas, colicky cramps, epigastric fullness, bloating, belching. The pulse tends to be wiry and the tongue appears greasy.

APPLICATION

Colic, indigestion, epigastric distension, gastrointestinal neurosis.

CONTRAINDICATION

Caution should be taken with the use of Smartweed.

Herbs and Actions
Chamomile and Fennel act as carminatives. Smartweed acts as a diuretic and diaphoretic. Licorice is a synergist and harmonizer.

Modification
Dill or Anise seed can be added to accentuate the carminative effect. Ginger can be added for nausea and vomiting. Peppermint can be added for throat irritation due to belching.

Commentary
This formula comes from Joseph Meyer's ***The Herbalist***. It is the only formula he recommended for children, and claimed that it was absolutely harmless to children.

Father John's Stomach Tea

Therapeutic Principle
Carminative.

Constituents
- Thousand Seal (*Achillea millefolium*)
- Juniper Berries (*Juniperis communis*)
- Milkweed (*Euphorbia corollata*)
- Blue Gentian (*Gentiana catesbaei*)
- Wormwood Leaves (*Artemesia vulgaris*)
- German Cheese Plant (*Malva rotundifolia*)
- Rose Pink (*Sabbatia angularis*)

Form
Tea.

Dosage
One cup three times per day.

Indication
Dyspepsia, indigestion, belching, bloating, abdominal pain. The tongue usually appears greasy and with teeth marks on the side. The pulse is either wiry or slippery.

Application
Indigestion, gastric and duodenal ulcers, chronic gastritis.

Contraindication
Contraindicated in pregnancy.

Herbs and Actions
Rose Pink acts as a bitter tonic in dyspepsia and convalescence. Milkweed acts a diaphoretic and epispastic. Yarrow acts as an aromatic tonic. Juniper acts as a stimulant and diuretic. Gentian is a bitter and stomachic. Cheeseplant acts as a demulcent and emollient. Wormwood is a tonic and appetite stimulant.

Modification
Chamomile can be added as a calming carminative. Geranium can be added in cases of ulcers.

Commentary
This old formula was recorded by Joseph Meyer in his herbal (1934). Yarrow acts as an aromatic tonic, but also can act as a hemostatic in cases of duodenal or gastric ulcers. Rose Pink can be tonifying to chronic, debilitating cases; spasm can be controlled by Milkweed.

Sassafras Compound

THERAPEUTIC PRINCIPLE

Carminative.

CONSTITUENTS

- Sassafras (*Sassafras albidum*)
- Elder Flowers (*Sambucus nigra*)
- Rosemary Leaves (*Rosemarinus officinalis*)
- Oregon Grape Root (*Mahonia aquafolia*)
- Chickweed (*Stellaria media*)
- Poke (*Phytolacca americana*)
- Horsetail (*Eqisetum arvense*)

FORM

Tea.

DOSAGE

One cup three times per day.

INDICATION

Dyspepsia, abdominal pain, belching, indigestion, bloating. The pulse can be wiry or slippery. The tongue usually appears greasy or slippery.

APPLICATION

Indigestion, gastric or duodenal ulcer, chronic gastritis, cholecystitis, mesenteric lymphadenopathy.

CONTRAINDICATION

Contraindicated in pregnancy.

Herbs and Actions
Sassafras acts an aromatic, alterative, and tonic. Elder acts as a stimulant. Rosemary also acts as a gentle stimulant. Poke Root moves the mesenteric lymphatic system, removing pain and swelling. Berberis acts as an astringent and stomachic, similar to the way Hydrastis does. Synergistically, the herbs act as a carminative, astringent, and tonic.

Modification
With bad breath, add Hydrastis. For pain in the hypochondrium, add Corydalis.

Commentary
This formula was recorded by Joseph Meyer in ***The Herbalist*** (1934). It is a serious carminative for long-standing painful conditions. Poke Root will move the mesenteric lymphatic system, removing pain. Sassafras acts as an alterative, returning metabolism back to normal.

Celery Angelica Compound

Therapeutic Principle
Carminative.

Constituents
- Celery Seed (*Apium graveolens*)
- Angelica Root (*Angelica archangelica*)
- Gentian Root (*Gentian lutea*)
- Sacred Bark (*Rhamnus purshiana*)
- Marshmallow Root (*Althea officinalis*)
- Bearberry Leaves (*Arctostaphylos uva-ursi*)
- Juniper Berries (*Juniperus communis*)
- German Cheese Plant (*Malva rotundifolia*)

Form
Decoction.

Dosage
One cup three times per day.

Indication
Indigestion, belching, hypochondriac pain, bloating and distension of the abdomen. The pulse is usually wiry, and the tongue usually appears greasy.

Application
Indigestion, chronic gastritis, duodenal ulcer, gastric ulcer, constipation.

Contraindication
Contraindicated in pregnancy.

Herbs and Actions
Cheeseplant acts as a demulcent and emollient. Juniper acts as a stimulant and diuretic. Bearberry acts as an astringent and tonic. Marshmallow acts as a demulcent and emollient. Sacred Bark acts as a laxative to excite peristalsis of the bowels. Gentian acts as a bitter tonic and stomachic. Angelica acts as carminative, stimulant, and aromatic. Celery acts as a carminative and appetizer (Meyer, 1934).

Modification
With portal congestion, add Collinsonia and Hydrastis (Priest, 1982).

Commentary
This is a carminative formula recorded by Joseph Meyer in his herbal (1934). Its design is to assist the entire body in elimination. Celery and Angelica are paired as carminatives. Cheese Plant and Marshmallow are paired as demulcents and emollients. Juniper and Bearberry assist as a pair in elimination through the kidneys and bladder. Sacred Bark aids in elimination through the bowels, while Gentian tonifies the digestive system.

Father Bernard's Stomach Tea

Therapeutic Principle
Carminative.

Constituents
- Italian Sage leaves (*Salvia officinalis*)
- Stone Root (*Collinsonia canadensis*)
- Colic Root (*Liatrus spicata*)
- Fennel Seed (*Foeniculum vulgare*)
- Wormwood leaves (*Artemesia vulgaris*)
- Gentian Root (*Gentian lutea*)
- Juniper Berries (*Juniperus communis*)
- Wild Strawberry Leaves (*Fragaria virginia*)
- German Cheese Plant (*Malva rotundifolia*)

Form
Decoction.

Dosage
Take one cup three times per day.

Indication
Indigestion, belching, bitter taste in mouth, chest pain, hypochondriac pain, constipation, throat dry, urine yellow. The pulse is usually wiry and rapid. The tongue is usually red with a yellow coating.

Application
Indigestion, hepatitis, hypertension, abdominal pain, genital itching, urethritis, acute cholecystitis, acute cystitis.

Contraindication
Contraindicated in pregnancy.

Herbs and Actions

This formula is a grouping of herbs that is valuable as a stomachic. The herbs act as stomach tonics, carminatives, and aid in the secretion of gastric juices. Strawberry acts as an astringent and tonic. Sage is of benefit to digestion and a weak tonic. Stone Root acts as a tonic. Colic Root acts as a bitter tonic. Cheese Plant acts as a demulcent. Wormwood acts as a carminative, stomachic, and cholagogue. Fennel acts as a carminative. Gentian acts as a stomachic, tonic, and cholagogue. Juniper acts as a carminative, stomachic and tonic.

Modification

For burning stomach pains, add Hydrastis and Berberis. For genital herpes, add Hyssop, Hypericum, and Melissa.

Commentary

This is a formula recorded by Joseph Meyer in his herbal (Meyer, 1934). It includes herbs that not only act as carminatives, but also tonify the stomach, stimulate hydrochloric acid production, act as cholagogues, demulcents, and assist with elimination through the kidneys and bladder.

Stamet's Carminative Formula

Therapeutic Principle

Carminative.

Constituents

- 1 part Anise (*Pimpinella anisum*)
- 1 part Fennel (*Foeniculum vulgare*)
- 1 part Caraway (*Carum carvi*)
- 1 part Coriander (*Coriandrum sativum*)

Form

Infusion.

Dosage

Take one cup three times per day.

INDICATION
Indigestion, bloating, abdominal pain, belching, flatulence. The pulse tends to be wiry and the tongue greasy.

APPLICATION
Indigestion, gastric ulcer, chronic gastritis.

CONTRAINDICATION
These herbs are all mild foods.

HERBS AND ACTIONS
Coriander acts as an anti-spasmodic, appetizer, carminative, and stomachic. The rest of the herbs act as carminatives and stomachics.

MODIFICATION
Add Hydrastis and Eupatorium for gastrointestinal flu.

COMMENTARY
This mild carminative is recorded in Zeanith Stamets (1954) book, ***Botanical Research and Treatment of Disease***. He was trained as a medical doctor, naturopath, chiropractor, and pharmacist. All of these herbs are foods, and show that some of our most effective herbs are gentle, nourishing food.

The Alterative/Blood Regulating Formulas

Use

- To invigorate blood circulation and remove stasis.
- To invigorate lymphatic circulation.
- As an anti-inflammatory.
- To increase monocytes and phagocytes.
- To regulate the immune system.
- To improve metabolism.

Formulas

Trifolium Compound/Hoxsey Formula

THERAPEUTIC PRINCIPLE

Blood purifier; invigorate the circulation; lymphatic and glandular alterative.

CONSTITUENTS

- 2 parts Red Clover Blossom (*Trifolium pratense*)
- 2 parts Licorice (*Glycyrriza glabra*)
- ½ part Buckthorn Bark (*Rhamnus frangula*)
- 1 part Burdock (*Arctium lappa*)
- 1 part Stillingia Root (*Stillingia sylvatica*)
- 1 part Oregon Grape Root (*Berberis aquifolium*)
- ½ part Phytolacca Root (*Phytolacca americana*)
- ½ part Prickly Ash Bark (*Xanthoxylum clava-herculis*)
- 1/8 part Wild Indigo Root (*Baptisia tinctoria*)
- Potassium Iodide USP

FORM

Decoction.

DOSAGE

Tea, three cups per day warm. Tincture, 30-60 drops three times per day.

INDICATION

Pain of a fixed nature, anorexia, wasting, glandular swelling, glandular congestion, loss of voice, sore throat, constipation, sinus pain and congestion, joint pain, pain in the ear, and moist, red, irritable skin, irritability. The pulse tends to be wiry, taut, and hesitant, while the tongue usually appears dark red with purple spots. The lymphatic rosary and radii solaris can be present in the iris.

APPLICATION

Cancer, tumors, swollen lymph nodes, sore throat, constipation, laryngitis, bronchitis, pharyngitis, arthritis, skin diseases, chronic middle ear infections, detoxification.

CONTRAINDICATION

Contraindicated in pregnancy and nursing mothers. Not to be taken for acute conditions associated with fever, inflammation, or infection (Smith, 1997).

Herbs and Actions

The herbs in this formula act as alteratives and blood purifiers. The formula's action is through the lymphatic, glandular and mucus membrane system, where it acts to alter disordered processes of the metabolic and catabolic humors, especially the elimination of metabolic waste (Smith, 1997). Red clover acts as an alterative and anti-cancer herb. Licorice acts as a demulcent and harmonizer. Buckthorn acts as a laxative. Burdock acts as an alterative, diaphoretic, and laxative. Stillingia acts as an alterative, with particular action on secretory and lymphatic functions, and is also anti-cancer. Oregon Grape Root acts as an alterative, lymphgogue, and anti-cancer herb. Prickly Ash acts as an alterative, tonic, and diaphoretic. Potassium iodide acts as an alterative and diuretic.

Modification

For amenorrhea and dysmenorrhea, add Mother's wort, Licorice, and Corydalis. For prostate cancer, add Saw Palmetto. For breast cancer, add Sheep Sorrel, Echinacea, and drop doses of Conium. Podophyllum can be added for more lymphatic work. Cascara can be added for a more purging action.

Commentary

The Trifolium/Hoxsey formula is a very popular and time proven remedy for some cancers. Many patients have made successful trips to the Hoxsey clinic in Mexico. Trifolium Compound was first recorded by Parke, Davis & Co. in 1890. It was considered one of the most valuable alteratives known, indicated for skin disorders, scrofulosis, and syphilis, and used as a tonic to the excretory, assimilative, and digestive organs. King's American Dispensatory listed it in 1898 as a tonic, alterative, and eliminative used for scrofula, chronic rheumatism, syphilis, and glandular and skin conditions (King, 1989). Harry Hoxsey made the formula famous by using it quite successfully with many cancers.

Scudder's Alterative

Therapeutic Principle

Alterative, lymphatic and glandular alterative, invigorate blood circulation.

Constituents

- 1 part Turkey Corn Root tincture (*Corydalis Formosa*)
- 1 part Yellow Dock Root tincture (*Rumex crispus*)
- 1 part Tag Alder Bark tincture (*Alnus serrulata*)
- 1 part Figwort Leaves/Root tincture (*Scrophularia nodosa*)
- 1 part Mayapple Root infusion (*Podophyllum peltatum*) (One ounce powder in four ounces boiling water; let sit two hours; strain)
- 1 part sugar (honey or syrup) dissolved in warm Podophyllum extract

Form

Tincture.

Dosage

Fifteen to twenty drops, two to three times per day, in water.

Indications

Liver congestion, pain of a fixed nature, glandular swelling, rashes, glandular congestion, irritability, insomnia. The pulse tends to be wiry. The tongue can be dark red.

Application

Liver congestion, swollen lymph nodes, skin disorders, arthritis, detoxification, constipation, cancer, tumors.

Contraindication

Contraindicated in pregnancy and nursing mothers.

Herbs and Actions

Turkey Corn acts as an alterative, tonic, anodyne, anti-cancer, and detoxicant. King (1898) said that it increases wastes and improves nutrition. Yellow Dock acts as an alterative, tonic, and blood purifier. Tag Alder acts as an alterative, increasing wastes and stimulating nutrition. Figwort acts as an alterative with particular affinity to the glandular system and the blood. Mayapple acts as a purgative, alterative, and cathartic.

Modification

Add Poke Root, False Bittersweet, Juniper Berries, Prickly Ash, and Guaiacum Wood to form Eli Jones' Cancer Syrup.

Notes

This famous cancer and liver alterative formula was developed by John Milton Scudder, MD, Professor of Materia Medica at the Eclectic Institute and author of ***Specific Diagnosis, Specific Medication***, and other textbooks. Of note is the method of extraction for this formula. Four of the herbs are tinctured, while Mayapple is an infusion. This changes it from more of a cathartic to an alterative action.

Turska's Formula

Therapeutic Principle

Regulate the blood, promote circulation, cleanse the blood, promote lymph movement.

Constituents

- 30 drops Aconite (*Aconitum napellus*)
- 30 drops Bryonia (*Bryonia Alba*)
- 30 drops Gelsemium (*Gelsemium sempervirens*)
- 1 drahm Phytolacca (*Phytolacca decandra*)
- 4 ounces Distilled water

Form

Tincture.

Dosage
One teaspoon four times daily.

Indication
Pain in the chest, pain in the abdomen, chronic hiccough, irritability, insomnia, emotional upset. The pulse tends to be wiry or hesitant. The tongue tends to be dark red with purple spots. The lymphatic rosary can be present in the iris.

Application
Uterine cysts, ovarian cysts, mammary cysts, fibrocystic breast disease, coronary heart disease, angina pectoris, cartilage costalgia, respiratory conditions, neuromusculoskeletal conditions.

Contraindication
This formula is composed of toxic botanicals and is for skilled professional use only. Contraindicated in pregnancy.

Herbs and Actions
The herbs in this formula are potent alteratives. Aconite increases the power of the heart, lessens the frequency of the pulses, removes obstruction to the flow of blood in the vessels, and antagonizes inflammatory action. It is indicated in mastitis and acute pain. Bryonia works with Gelsemium and Aconite on the nervous system, relieving neuralgias. Gelsemium reduces autonomic nervous system irritability and pain. Phytolacca acts as an alterative and lymphagogue.

Modifications
For amenorrhea and dysmenorrhea, add Leonurus.

Commentary
This formula was given to us by Dr. Turska, a naturopathic physician who linked the old naturopaths to the contemporary era. It has also been called the cyst formula due to its ability to help reduce uterine, ovarian, and mammary cysts (Boyle, 1993).

Essiac Tea

Therapeutic Principle

Invigorate the blood circulation and remove blood stasis.

Constituents

- 52 parts Burdock Root (*Arctium lappa*)
- 16 parts Sheep Sorrel (*Rumex acetosella*)
- 1 part Turkey Rhubarb (*Rheum palmatum*)
- 4 parts Slippery Elm (*Ulmus fulva*)

Form

Decoction.

Dosage

Take four tablespoons or two ounces once in the morning, five minutes before eating, and once in the evening, at least two hours after eating. As a preventative, take daily four tablespoons or two ounces at bedtime or on an empty stomach at least two hours after eating.

Indication

Pain, chronic pain of a fixed and piercing nature, abdominal pain, pain with hardening, lumps, irritability, indigestion, constipation, insomnia, emotional upset. The tongue tends to be purple with spots on the side or dark red with purple spots. The pulse is usually wiry and taut, with a hesitancy. The lymphatic rosary and radii solaris can be present in the iris.

Application

Detoxification, cancer, AIDS, chronic fatigue, lupus, alzheimers, multiple sclerosis, chronic pain, coronary heart disease, tumors, anorexia.

Contraindication

Contraindicated in pregnancy.

Herbs and Actions

Sheep sorrel and Burdock are the emperor herbs that act to destroy cancer. The Slippery Elm and Rhubarb assist by increasing bile flow and assisting the intestinal tract to eliminate the toxins released by the formula (Percival, 1994).

Modification

There is an optional modification of the formula, where is added 2 parts Kelp, 1 part Red Clover, 1 part Blessed Thistle, and 0.4 parts Watercress. This tends to enhance the effectiveness of the formula if directed to the thyroid gland and liver detoxification and blood purification (Percival, 1994).

Commentary

This very popular formula for cancer was handed down by an Ojibway herbalist to Rene Caisse (Essiac is Caisse spelled backwards), a Canadian nurse who treated many terminal cancer patients successfully.

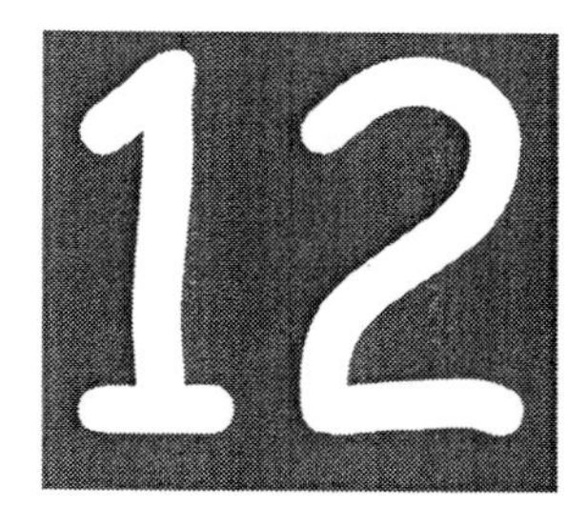

The Diuretic Formulas

Use

- To increase the rate of urine flow.
- To increase glomerular filtration or decreased tubular reabsorption.
- To increase the excretion of sodium.
- As an antiviral, antifungal, or antibacterial.

Formulas

Diuretic Syrup

THERAPEUTIC PRINCIPLE
Diuretic.

CONSTITUENTS
- 4 ounces Queen of the Meadow (*Eupatorium purpureum*)
- 4 ounces Juniper Berries (*Juniperis communis*)
- 4 ounces Cleavers (*Galium aparine*)
- 4 ounces Burdock root or seed (*Arctium lappa*)

FORM
Syrup.

Dosage

Take half a glass three times per day (Colby, 1846). To prepare, make a strong decoction, strain and add two pounds of honey and half as much gin as there is of the tea. Bottle for use (Colby, 1846).

Indication

Edema, dizziness, shortness of breath, cough, diarrhea, difficulty in urination. The pulse is usually superficial and rapid. The tongue usually appears white and slippery.

Application

Gravel, strangury, dropsy, edema, cardiac edema, chronic nephritic edema, diarrhea.

Contraindication

Contraindicated in pregnancy. Should not be used for over six weeks.

Herbs and Actions

The herbs act synergistically as cooling diuretics. Queen of the Meadow acts as a relaxant, diuretic, antilithic, and has an affinity to the kidneys and bladder. Juniper acts as an antiseptic, diuretic, stomachic, and tonic. Cleavers acts as a diuretic and soothing relaxant to the kidneys and bladder. Burdock acts as an alterative, diuretic, and powerful blood purifier.

Modification

With indigestion, diarrhea, and decreased urination, add Cinnamon. With jaundice and dysuria, add Wormwood.

Commentary

This formula is from Samuel Thomson and was recorded by Benjamin Colby (1846) is his book ***A Guide to Health***. Dr. Colby was a student of Samuel Thomson's. This formula has a strong alterative action with the addition of Burdock. Although diuresis is our main action, we must also assist all of the other organs of the body.

Formula for Bright's Disease

Therapeutic Principle
Diuretic.

Constituents
- 1 part Juniper Berries (*Juniperis communis*)
- 1 part Blue Cohosh (*Caulophyllum thalictroides*)
- 1 part Couchgrass (*Agropyron repens*)
- 1 part Buchu (*Barosma betulina*)

Form
Decoction.

Dosage
Take one-half cup three times per day.

Indication
Edema, dysuria, cough, shortness of breath, spitting saliva. The pulse is usually superficial, and the tongue usually appears white and slippery.

Application
Bright's disease, edema, cardiac edema, chronic nephritic edema, ascites due to liver cirrhosis, urinary retention.

Contraindication
Contraindicated in pregnancy.

Herbs and Actions
The herbs act together as diuretics. Juniper acts as an antiseptic, diuretic, stomachic, and tonic. Blue Cohosh promotes diuresis and tonifies the kidneys. Couchgrass acts as a diuretic, tonic, demulcent, and emollient. Buchu acts as a nervine and tonic to the kidneys and bladder.

Modification
With liver disease, add Dandelion. With jaundice and dysuria, add Wormwood.

Commentary
This formula is from Dr. Christopher. He was a graduate of Dr. Nowell's Dominion Herbal College in Canada. Dr. Nowell's curriculum was based on Dr. Lyle's work, who was a student of Dr. Cook, the Physio-medicalist (Bergner, 2002). Physio-medicalism evolved out of Thomsonian Herbal Medicine. Dr. Christopher taught many modern herbalists, thus keeping a lineage going straight back to Thomsonian Herbalism.

Weiss' Diuretic Tea

Therapeutic Principles
Diuretic.

Constituents
- Juniper Fruit (*Juniperis communis*)
- Parsley Fruit (*Petroselinum satium*)
- Equisetum Herb (*Equisetum arvense*)
- Ononis Root (*Ononis spinosa*)
- Fennel Fruit (*Foeniculum vulgare*)
- Peppermint Leaves (*Mentha piperita*)

Form
Infusion.

Dosage
Take three cups daily, one to two teaspoons of herb per cup of boiling water, infuse for 20 minutes.

Indication
Edema, dysuria, cough, cholera, headache, palpitation below the umbilicus. The pulse tends to be superficial, and the tongue usually appears white and slippery.

Application

Cardiac edema, chronic nephritic edema, acute gastritis, acute enteritis.

Contraindication

Contraindicated in pregnancy.

Herbs and Actions

The herbs act synergistically as diuretics. Juniper acts as an antiseptic, diuretic, stomachic and tonic. Parsley acts as a diuretic and tonic. Equisetum directs the action of the herbs to the kidneys and bladder. Ononis acts as a gentle diuretic. Fennel acts as a diuretic, antispasmodic, aromatic, stimulant, and stomachic. Peppermint acts as a tonic, carminative, refrigerant, anodyne, cholagogue, stomachic, and anti-spasmodic.

Modification

For diarrhea and decreased urine, add Cinnamon. With cardiac involvement, add Mother's Wort.

Commentary

This formula is from the German medical herbalist Rudolf Weiss. He wrote a tremendous text on medical herbalism, ***Herbal Medicine***. It is based on the German scientific tradition. This formula has a more cooling effect to irritated and inflamed tissues with the addition of Peppermint. According to Weiss, "The best way of composing a diuretic tea is to combine one or two diuretics containing volatile oils, one or two with saponins, and finally one or two herbs that improve flavor and improve gastric tolerance (Weiss, 1988)."

Nephritis Formula

Therapeutic Principle

Diuretic.

CONSTITUENTS

- ½ ounce Uva Ursi (*Arctostaphylos uva-ursi*)
- ½ ounce Cleavers (*Galium aparine*)
- ½ ounce Juniper Berries (*Juniperus communis*)
- ½ ounce Marshmallow (*Althea officinalis*)
- ½ ounce Buchu (*Barosma betulina*)
- 1 teaspoon Cayenne (*Capsicum minimum*)

FORM

Decoction.

DOSAGE

One cup three times per day.

INDICATION

Water retention, fever, thirst, headache, vomiting, diarrhea. The pulse tends to be superficial and rapid. The tongue usually appears slippery.

APPLICATION

Edema, difficult urination, cough, shortness of breath, headache, nephritis.

CONTRAINDICATION

Contraindicated in pregnancy.

HERBS AND ACTIONS

Marshmallow acts as a soothing demulcent. Uva Ursi acts as a diuretic and tonic. Cleavers acts as a diuretic and soothing relaxant to the kidneys and bladder. Juniper acts as an antiseptic, diuretic, stomachic, and tonic. Marshmallow acts as a demulcent to soothe the urinary tract. Buchu acts as a nervine and tonic, chiefly influencing the bladder and increasing the flow of urine. Cayenne acts as a stimulant and synergist.

MODIFICATION

Administer with a tea made of Slippery Elm.

Commentary

This formula is recorded in Dr. Christopher's herbal (1976). He was a graduate of Dr. Nowell's Dominion Herbal College in Canada. Dr. Nowell's curriculum was based on Dr. Lyle's work, who was a student of Dr. Cook, the Physio-medicalist (Bergner, 2002). Physio-medicalism evolved out of Thomsonian Herbal Medicine. Dr. Christopher taught many modern herbalists, thus keeping a lineage going straight back to Thomsonian Herbalism.

Venetian Herb Tea for Children

Therapeutic Principle

Diuretic.

Constituents

- Bearberry Leaves (*Arctostaphylos uva-ursi*)
- Cheese Plant (*Althea officinalis*)
- Corn Silk (*Zea mays*)
- Sassafras Root Bark (*Sassafras albidum*)
- St. John's Wort (*Hypericum perforatum*)
- Horsetail Grass (*Equisetum arvense*)

Form

Infusion.

Dosage

Take one-half cup per day.

Indication

Enuresis, fever, thirst, headache, diarrhea. The pulse is usually superficial and rapid, and the tongue usually appears slippery. Nerve rings can be present in the iris.

Application

Enuresis, nephritis, water retention, headache.

Contraindication
Contraindicated in pregnancy.

Herbs and Actions
The Sassafras acts as a diaphoretic and taste enhancer. Bearberry and Horsetail direct their action toward the bladder and kidneys. Corn Silk helps with enuresis. St. John's Wort acts as a nervine. Cheese plant is soothing to the genito-urinary tract.

Modification
With jaundice and dysuria, add Wormwood.

Commentary
This formula was recorded by Joseph Meyer in his pocket herbal in 1918. It is good for children and has a mild and pleasant taste.

Father John's Compound

Therapeutic Principle
Diuretic.

Constituents
- Hepatica (*Hepatica triloba*)
- Seven Barks (*Hydrangea arborescens*)
- Chicory Root (*Cichorium intybus*)
- Senna (*Cassia marilandica*)
- Red Clover (*Trifolium pratense*)
- Boneset (*Eupatorium perfoliatum*)
- German Cheese Plant (*Althea officinalis*)
- Sassafras (*Sassafras albidum*)

Form
Decoction.

Dosage
One cup three times per day.

Indication
Water retention, fever, onset of cold, headache. The pulse tends to be superficial and rapid. The tongue usually appears slippery.

Application
Edema, cough, shortness of breath, influenza, nephritis.

Contraindication
Contraindicated in pregnancy.

Herbs and Actions
This is a very mild diuretic, stimulating the functions of elimination through bowels and urine (Meyer, 1934). Hepatica acts as a diuretic and helps move liver congestion. Seven barks acts as an antilithic and diuretic. Chicory acts as a diuretic, tonic, digestive, and cholagogue. Senna acts as a diuretic and cathartic. Red Clover acts as an alterative. Boneset acts as a tonic and mild laxative. Cheese Plant acts as a demulcent and emollient, soothing an irritated and inflamed urinary tract. Sassafras acts as a diuretic, antiseptic, and alterative.

Contraindication
Contraindicated with loose stools.

Modifications
With diarrhea, remove Senna and Boneset. With cardiac involvement, add Mother's Wort.

Commentary
This formula was recorded by Joseph Meyer in his herbal. It is a well-rounded diuretic formula, working on different organs within the body. Most of the herbs have a diuretic action, but they are assisted in different areas. Seven Barks acts also as an antilithic, with Cheese Plant soothing any inflamed or irritated portions of the urinary tract. Hepatica and Chicory help to move liver congestion and act as a cholagogue, assisting diuresis. Red Clover and Sassafras act as alteratives, gently assisting the entire healing process. Senna and Boneset move the bowels, assisting complete elimination. Boneset and Chicory are tonifying to the entire body.

Diuretic Beer

THERAPEUTIC PRINCIPLE
Diuretic.

CONSTITUENTS
- ½ pound Dandelion Roots (*Taraxacum officinale*)
- ½ pound Dandelion Tops (*Taraxacum officinale*)
- ½ pound Parsley Roots (*Petroselinum sativum*)
- ½ pound Parsley Tops (*Petroselinum sativum*)
- ½ pound Peach Leaves (*Prunus persica*)
- ½ pound Broom Tops (*Cytisus scoparius*)
- ½ pound Strawberry Leaves (*Fragaria vesca*)
- 2 ounces Juniper Berries (*Juniperus communis*)
- 1 pound Sugar

FORM
Beer.

DOSAGE
Take one cup three times per day. To prepare, boil the herbs in six quarts of water, strain and add the two ounces of pulverized Juniper berries and sugar. Balm and let it foment, then bottle in six hours (Simmonite, 1957).

INDICATION
Retention of water, thirst, edema, vomiting, difficulty in urination, cough, shortness of breath, diarrhea, palpitation below the umbilicus, cholera, dysuria.

APPLICATION
Chronic nephritic edema, cardiac edema, urinary retention, acute gastritis.

CONTRAINDICATION
Contraindicated in pregnancy. Parsley is contraindicated in acute kidney inflammations (Lust, 1974).

Herbs and Actions

Dandelion Roots act as a diuretic and promote the formation of bile. Dandelion Tops act as a diuretic, stomachic, and tonic. Parsley Roots act as a tonic and diuretic. Parsley Tops act as a diuretic. Peach Leaves act as a diuretic. Broom Tops act as a diuretic and cardiac stimulant. Strawberry Leaves act as a diuretic. Juniper Berries act as an antiseptic, diuretic, stomachic, and tonic.

Modifications

Add Hawthorne with cardiac conditions.

Commentary

This formula is recorded in ***The Simmonite-Culpeper Herbal*** (1957). It is a collection of herbs and formulas used by Dr. W. J. Simmonite and Nicolas Culpeper, a famed apothecary-physician-astrologer from the early 19th century. Culpeper's Herbal is still popular today. He felt that the only way to know how an herb functioned was astrologically. His herbal assigns each herb with an astrological house, and he would prescribe herbs from the house opposite the one that caused the disease, or sympathetically, within each house curing its own disease (Griggs, 1981).

Dr. Carroll's Kidney Formula

Therapeutic Principle

Diuretic.

Constituents

- 2 parts Marjoram (*Origanum vulgare*)
- 1 part Elder (*Sambucus canadensis*)

Form

Capsule.

Dosage

One to two capsules three times per day with warm water.

Indication
Edema, swelling of feet, legs, hands, arms; diarrhea, dysuria, vomiting, dizziness, cough, shortness of breath, thirst, headache, difficulty urinating. The pulse tends to be superficial and rapid; the tongue tends to have a white coating and appear slippery.

Application
Edema, chronic nephritic edema, acute gastritis, urinary retention, ascites due to liver cirrhosis.

Contraindication
None known.

Herbs and Actions
Elder is the chief herb that acts as a strong diuretic and alterative. Marjoram has a soothing action on the renal tissue.

Modification
For cardiac involvement, add 2 parts Mother's wort.

Commentary
This formula was introduced by Dr. O.G. Carroll as a diuretic formula to be used in cases of edema. The naturopathic approach to herbalism is evident in the inclusion of Elder as the chief herb with its alterative effect. The Marjoram harmonizes and soothes the strong diuretic action of the Elder.

Dr. Carroll's Edema Formula

Therapeutic Principle
Diuretic.

Constituents
- 2 parts Mother's wort (*Leonorus cardiaca*)
- 2 parts Dwarf Elder (*Sambucus ebulus*)
- 1 part Buchu (*Barosma betulina*)

Form
Capsule.

Dosage
1-2 capsules three times per day.

Indication
Edema, diarrhea, headache, difficulty urinating, cough, shortness of breath, palpitation, retention of fluid in the body, dysuria, vomiting, backache, chronic bladder ache and weakness, spitting saliva, indigestion, abdominal pain. The tongue tends to have a white and slippery coat, while the pulse is usually deep and thready.

Application
Edema, cardiac edema, congestive heart failure, chronic nephritis, hypothyroidism, rheumatoid arthritis, ascites.

Contraindication
Buchu is contraindicated in any case of acute or subacute irritation, as it is too simulating for such conditions (Cook, 1869).

Herbs and Actions
The Elder acts as a strong diuretic tonic and alterative, while the Mother's wort focuses the action on the heart. Buchu acts as a nervine and tonic, chiefly influencing the bladder and increasing the flow of urine.

Modification
With increased peritoneal fluid and shortness of brea th, Plantago Seed and Phytolacca root can be added. With symptoms of a more cold nature with diarrhea, Ginger can be added. For ascites, add Fraxinus, Button-snake root, and Cimicifuga.

Commentary
This formula from Dr. O. G. Carroll, a pillar in the modern Naturopathic community, changes the focus of the diuretic to include affecting the function of the heart.

13

The Anti-convulsant Formulas

Use

- For epilepsy, grand mal or petit mal.
- For spasms, dizziness, and convulsions.
- As an anti-hypertensive, anti-convulsant, anti-epileptic, sedative, or hypnotic in action.

Formulas

Antispasmodic Tincture

THERAPEUTIC PRINCIPLE
Antispasmodic and Anti-convulsant.

CONSTITUENTS
- 1 ounce Lobelia Seed (*Lobelia inflata*) granulated
- 1 ounce Skunk Cabbage (*Symplocarpus foetidus*) granulated
- 1 ounce Skullcap (*Scutellaria lateriflora*) granulated
- 1 ounce Black Cohosh (*Cimicifuga racemosa*) granulated
- 1 ounce Myrrh (*Commiphora myrrha*) granulated
- ½ ounce Cayenne (*Capsicum frutescens*) powdered
- 1 pint apple cider vinegar

Form

Tincture. Steep the herbs in one pint of water just below the boiling point for ½ hour. Strain, add the apple cider vinegar, and bottle (Kloss, 1939).

Dosage

For acute symptoms, take 30-40 drops in water three to five times per day. As a preventative or restorative tonic, take 15-30 drops in water two to three times per day (Smith, 1997).

Indication

Convulsions, spasms, spasmodic coughs, seizures, swelling, cramps, coma, headache, stiff neck, vertigo, trembling movement of the tongue, insomnia, deviation of the mouth and eyes, hemiplegia, restlessness. The tongue tends to be red, maybe with a yellow coating and dry. The pulse tends to be wiry, taut, and rapid.

Application

Spasms of any nature, hypertension, puerperal eclampsia, trigeminal neuralgia, convulsion, epilepsy, mania with convulsion, delirium tremors, fainting, childbirth, spasmodic croup, cramps, whooping cough, asthma, lockjaw, hydrophobia, lumbago, rheumatism, childbirth (Kloss, 1939; Smith, 1997).

Contraindication

Contraindicated with low blood pressure, and in individuals with low vitality and a weak constitution (Smith, 1997). If nausea or vomiting occur, discontinue use for 1-2 days and resume with a lower number of drops (Smith, 1997).

Herbs and Actions

The herbs in the formula act synergistically as an antispasmodic. Lobelia acts as a nervine, relaxant, and anti-spasmodic. Skunk Cabbage acts as an anti-spasmodic and relaxant. Skullcap acts as a nervine, relaxant, anti-spasmodic, and nervous system tonic. Black Cohosh acts as a relaxant, anti-spasmodic, and nervous system tonic. Myrrh acts as a stimulant to circulation and digestion. Cayenne acts as a stimulant and as a pair with Lobelia to secure an anti-spasmodic action.

Modification

With hypertensive headache and dizziness, add Gentian and Self-heal. With headache and vertigo, add Self-heal and Chrysanthemum flower. For more of an antispasmodic effect, add Lady's Slipper or Valerian.

Commentary

This popular formula was made famous by Jethro Kloss in his book, ***Back to Eden*** (1939). Jethro Kloss was a minister and was trained at the Battle Creek Sanitarium. He ran sanitariums throughout the country. His herbal influence is from the Physio-Medicalist and Thomsonian schools of Medical Herbalism. This formula is a modification of Samuel Thomson's anti-spasmodic tincture, also called Thomson's Third Preparation of Lobelia. Kloss used the Anti-spasmodic Tincture both internally and externally. Internally, it could be taken for cramps in the bowels, snake bites, pyorrhea, tonsillitis, and diptheria. Externally he would apply it to any muscle cramp, swelling, rheumatism, lumbago, and lockjaw (Kloss, 1939).

Thomson's Third Preparation of Lobelia/Thomson's Antispasmodic Tincture

Therapeutic Principle

Anti-spasmodic and Anti-convulsant.

Constituents

- ½ ounce Lobelia (*Lobelia inflata*)
- ½ ounce Capsicum (*Capsicum frutescens*)
- 2 drachms Lady's Slippers (*Cypripedium*)
- 8 ounces Compound Tincture of Myrrh
  - 1 pound Myrrh (*Commiphora myrrha*)
  - 1 ounce Capsicum (*Capsicum frutescens*)
  - 1 Gallon 85% Alcohol

Form

Tincture.

Dosage

"It may be used in doses of a teaspoonful, or much more, in water or some demulcent infusion, when vomiting is required under circumstances of depression – as in narcotic poisoning, apoplexy from overeating, membranous croup when Lobelia alone will make no impression, etc. It is to be given at short intervals, so as to obtain very prompt action. In sudden depression of the pulse, all forms of collapse, and shock of injury, it is unequaled as a stimulant; and may be given in doses ranging from a few drops to one or two teaspoonsful, every five or ten minutes, till reaction is obtained (Cook, 1869)."

Indication

Convulsions, spasms, spasmodic coughs, seizures, swelling, cramps, coma, headache, stiff neck, vertigo, trembling movement of the tongue, insomnia, deviation of the mouth and eyes, hemiplegia, restlessness. The tongue tends to be red, maybe with a yellow coating and dry. The pulse tends to be wiry, taut, and rapid.

Application

Spasms of any nature, hypertension, puerperal eclampsia, trigeminal neuralgia, convulsion, epilepsy, mania with convulsion, delirium tremors, fainting, childbirth, spasmodic croup, cramps, whooping cough, asthma, lockjaw, hydrophobia, lumbago, rheumatism, childbirth (Kloss, 1939; Smith, 1997).

Contraindication

Contraindicated with low blood pressure, and in individuals with low vitality and a weak constitution (Smith, 1997). If nausea or vomiting occur, discontinue use for one to two days and resume with a lower number of drops (Smith, 1997).

Herbs and Actions

Lobelia acts as a nervine, relaxant, and antispasmodic. Capsicum acts as a stimulant and as a pair with Lobelia to secure an antispasmodic action. Lady's Slippers acts as a relaxant, nervine, parodyne, and antispasmodic. Myrrh acts as a stimulant to circulation and digestion, and works as a pair with Capsicum.

Modifications

Remove the Compound Tincture of Myrrh and increase the Lady's Slippers to ½ ounce and we have Dr. Wilkinson's Anti-spasmodic Drops. Remove the Compound Tincture of Myrrh and add Blue Cohosh and Anise Seeds and we have Dr. Cook's Anti-spasmodic Drops. Both of these modifications are less stimulating (Cook, 1869).

Commentary

This is the original Anti-spasmodic Tincture developed by Dr. Samuel Thomson, also called Thomson's Third Preparation of Lobelia and Compound Tincture of Lobelia and Capsicum. Dr. Cook said that "It is probably the most powerful stimulating and relaxing compound ever devised, making its impression with wonderful force, and extending through the system, as Dr. Thomson well remarks, 'like electricity' (Cook, 1869)." Cook said that it will powerfully arouse the stomach, nervous system, and circulations, and that it is the most efficient anti-spasmodic.

Dr. Rudgley's Formula for Paralysis

Therapeutic Principle

Anti-spasmodic and anti-convulsant.

Constituents

- 4 handfuls Wood Betony (*Betonica officinalis*)
- 1 handful Rosemary (*Rosmarinus officinalis*)
- 1 handful Sage (*Salvia officinalis*)
- 2 pounds Juniper Berries (*Juniperus communis*)
- 24 grams Senna, Powder (*Cassia angustifolia; Cassia acutifolia*)
- 24 grams Ginger (*Zingiber officinale*)
- 15 grams Cubebs (*Piper cubeba*)
- 2 pounds Sugar
- 15 grams Sweet Flag (*Acorus calamus*) (Christopher,1976)

Form

Tea.

Dosage
One tablespoon morning and night. To prepare, simmer the first three herbs slowly in one gallon of water down to ½ gallon. Strain, add the sugar, bring to a boil, and remove the surface scum. Strain hot over the other herbs, cover tightly until cool and then strain (Christopher, 1976).

Indication
Paralysis, inability to control body movement, deviation of the eyes and mouth, tinnitis, vertigo, distension in the eyes, dizziness, unconsciousness, coma. The pulse tends to be wiry, and the tongue appears red usually.

Application
Apoplexy, epilepsy, apoplectiform, glaucoma.

Contraindication
Contraindicated in pregnancy.

Herbs and Actions
Wood Betony acts as a nervine and tonic. Rosemary acts as a relaxant, nervine, and anti-spasmodic. Sage acts as a nervine and relaxant. Juniper acts as a strengthener of the brain, memory, and optic nerve. Senna acts as both a relaxant and a stimulating cathartic. Ginger works as an aromatic pair to Senna, relieving the gripping effect of Senna that is often very unpleasant to nervous temperaments (Cook, 1869). Cubebs stimulate the kidneys and bladder and acts as a sedative. Sweet Flag acts as a relaxant, aromatic, and assists with atonic dyspepsia.

Modification
For bitter taste in the mouth and red face, add Wormwood. For headache and vertigo, add Self-Heal.

Commentary

The preparation of this formula is important, particularly the first three herbs, in order to extract the important constituents to act as nervines (Cook, 1869). Some of the other herbs are aromatic, which open the orifices of the head, and their aromatic principles must be retained, hence only an infusion is prepared from them. This is a well-constructed formula. Paralysis can affect digestion, the bowels and kidneys. We have nervines and anti-spasmodic herbs, but they are combined with digestives, herbs to move the bowels, and herbs to move the kidneys. Aromatic herbs, such as Ginger, Cubebs, and Sweet Flag are used to both open the orifices (senses) and dampen the cathartic effect of Senna on someone with a nervous disorder.

Dr. Christopher's Epilepsy Formula

Therapeutic Principle

Anti-spasmodic and anti-convulsant.

Constituents

- ½ ounce Skullcap (*Scutellaria lateriflora*)
- ½ ounce Wood Betony (*Betonica officinalis*)
- ¼ ounce Valerian root (*Valeriana officinalis*)
- ½ ounce Pennyroyal (*Hedeoma pulegioides*)
- ½ ounce Centaury (*Erythraea centaurium*)
- ½ teaspoonful Cayenne (*Capsicum minimum*)
- ½ teaspoonful Bayberry bark (*Myrica cerifera*)

Form

Tea.

Dosage

Two tablespoons six times daily. To prepare, infuse the first five herbs in one quart of water. Cover closely and keep warm in the oven for one hour, then strain over the Cayenne and Bayberry. Sweeten with honey, bottle, and keep in a cool place.

INDICATION

Epilepsy, convulsions, spasms. The pulse tends to be wiry and the tongue usually appears red. Nerve rings tend to be present in the iris.

APPLICATION

Epilepsy, paralysis, convulsions.

CONTRAINDICATION

Contraindicated in pregnancy.

HERBS AND ACTIONS

The herbs act synergistically as an anti-convulsant. Skullcap is the key herb in this formula; it is a powerful nervine and anti-spasmodic. The Wood Betony is again used in another anti-convulsant, acting as a nervine. The Valerian is another traditionally used nervine; it also has a mild stimulating effect as an anti-spasmodic and it is soothing to the nervous system. Pennyroyal also has a soothing and relaxing effect to the nervous system. Cayenne and Bayberry are used as stimulants in this formula.

COMMENTARY

This is one of Dr. Christopher's formulas for epilepsy. Dr. Christopher studied at Dominion Herbal College, where the curriculum was written by Dr. Nowell, who was influenced by Dr. Lyle, a student of Dr. Cook. This gives us our lineage back to Dr. Samuel Thomson. According to Dr. Christopher, "Skullcap is one of the best nervine agents that nature provides...it is as stimulating as quinine...[and] is an excellent anti-spasmodic agent (Christopher, 1976)."

14

The Moisturizing Formulas

Use

- To moisturize the body.
- To moisturize the lungs.
- To treat dryness and chronic dehydration.

Formulas

Tuberculosis Formula

THERAPEUTIC PRINCIPLE
Moisturize; eliminate dryness in the lung.

Constituents

- 1 ounce Elecampane root (*Inula helenium*)
- 3 ounces Comfrey root (*Symphytum officinalis*)
- 1 ounce Horehound (*Marrubium vulgare*)
- 1 ounce Licorice root (*Glycyrrhiza glabra*)
- 1 ounce Iceland moss (*Venraria islandica*)
- ½ ounce Peruvian bark (*Cinchona calisaya*)
- ¼ ounce Composition powder
- ¼ teaspoon Cayenne (*Capsicum minimum*)
- 3 ounces Acacia (*Acacia senegal*)
- 1 pound Sugar
- 1 ounce Queen's delight, tincture (*Stillingia sylvatica*)
- 1 ounce Antispasmodic tincture

Form

Tea.

Dosage

The first week drink one wineglassful five to six times daily. The second and third weeks increase gradually to eight times daily (Christopher, 1976). To prepare, simmer the first seven herbs in three quarts of water down to two quarts. Strain hot over the Cayenne and dissolve in the Acacia and sugar. To each 14 ounces, add the given amount of Queen's Delight and antispasmodic tincture. Administer with one-half pint of Slippery Elm gruel in the morning and evening. Also drink Slippery Elm and lemon drink (Christopher, 1976).

Indication

Cough, cough with blood, dry and painful throat, cough and asthma with bloody sputum, heat sensation in the hands and feet, fever, dryness in the nose and lips, wheezing. The tongue is usually red, with little coating. The pulse tends to be rapid and thready or weak.

Application

Tuberculosis, tuberculosis with severe hemorrhage, hemoptysis, cough, asthma.

Contraindication

Contraindicated for a patient with cough due to excess phlegm.

Herbs and Actions

Elecampane is strengthening to the lungs, acting as an astringent and tonic. Comfrey acts as a soothing tonic and mucilage. Horehound has a great affinity for the lungs, acting as an expectorant, tonic, and stimulant. Licorice acts as a demulcent and relaxant, and is soothing to mucus irritations. Iceland Moss acts as a demulcent and tonic. Peruvian Bark acts as an anti-periodic and nervous system tonic. Composition Powder acts as a stimulant and astringent. Cayenne acts as a stimulant, particularly on circulation and the nervous system. Acacia acts as a mucilage, demulcent, and nutritive. Queen's Delight acts as a stimulant to the glands, bowels, and circulation. Anti-spasmodic Tincture acts as an anti-spasmodic, stimulant, and relaxant. It arouses the vital force and stimulates the nervous system.

Modification

For diphtheria, add Goldenseal, Honeysuckle flower, and Mint. With inflammation and swelling of the throat, add Violet and Dandelion. For tuberculosis with cavity, add Agrimony. If sweat is present, remove Composition powder. Blue Cohosh and Anise Seed can be added to enhance the anti-spasmodic effects with a prostrated patient.

Commentary

This formula's roots go back to Dr. Samuel Thomson. It is a classic example of how two smaller formulas are combined to form a third formula with a different action. In this formula, Composition Powder and Anti-spasmodic Tincture are combined with more nourishing herbs in order to make a different formula with a specific purpose. This formula is recorded by Dr. Christopher, a medical herbalist who linked the modern herbalist to traditional herbalism, with roots back into the Thomsonian and Physio-Medicalist Traditions.

Dr. Coffin's Consumption Formula

THERAPEUTIC PRINCIPLE
Moisturizing formula.

CONSTITUENTS
- ½ ounce Raspberry Leaves (*Rubus idaeus*)
- ½ ounce Agrimony (*Agrimonia eupatoria*)
- ½ ounce Barberry Bark (*Berberis vulgaris*)
- ½ ounce Cleavers (*Galium aparine*)
- ½ ounce Ground Ivy (*Glechoma hederacea*)
- ½ ounce European Centaury (*Erythraea centauria*)
- ½ ounce Horehound (*Marrubium vulgare*)
- ½ teaspoon Cayenne (*Capsicum minimum*)
- ¼ ounce Licorice (*Glycyrrhiza glabra*)

FORM
Decoction.

DOSAGE
Take one cup three times per day.

INDICATION
Cough, asthma, heat sensation in body, diarrhea. The pulse tends to be thready and rapid. The tongue usually appears red with little coating.

APPLICATION
Tuberculosis, cough, asthma, hemoptysis, diarrhea, cholera.

CONTRAINDICATION
Contraindicated with a patient with common cold and excess symptoms.

Herbs and Actions

Raspberry acts as a mild and soothing astringent, slightly tonifying. Agrimony acts as a stimulant and astringent. Barberry acts as a tonic, stimulating appetite and strength in debilitated conditions, and also acts as a hepatic. Cleavers is soothing to the nervous system and acts as a soothing relaxant on the kidneys and bladder. Ground Ivy is an expectorant and tonic to the lungs. Centaury acts as a tonic and digestive. Horehound acts as an expectorant, tonic, and stimulant. Cayenne equalizes circulation and prevents a fatal collapse. Licorice acts as a demulcent and soothes mucus and bronchial irritations.

Modifications

Add Ginger for a more warming effect and to stimulate circulation more.

Commentary

This formula is from one of the great herbalists of the 19th century. Dr. Albert Isaiah Coffin was first trained in conventional medicines as an apprentice until his own illness didn't respond (he claimed to expectorate three pints of matter a day and sometimes a pint of blood), at which time a Seneca Indian woman cured him with an herbal decoction that caused a sensation of "a comfortable, flow diffusing itself over my whole frame...a pleasant moisture bedewed my hands and I felt as one reprieved from a sentence of death (Coffin, 1866)." He then studied with the Seneca, until learning of Dr. Samuel Thomson and studying his patented herbal medicine system. At age 48, Dr. Coffin brought his botanic system to England and created quite a stir. He was successful in treating cholera by wrapping his patients warmly and applying a hot brick at their feet, giving liberal amounts of herbal decoctions to counter dehydration, and replenishing potassium and alkaline losses, giving astringent rectal injections, and normalizing circulation with Cayenne and Ginger (Griggs, 1981).

The Sedative or Tranquilizing Formulas

Use

- As sedatives to calm or induce sleeping (sleep is a state of rest and repair).
- As a tranquilizer (implies mental calmness without depression of mental activity).
- As nourishing sedatives.
- To improve the integrity, mental spirit, and thinking process of the brain.

Formulas

Nervine Capsules

THERAPEUTIC PRINCIPLE
Sedative with a nourishing effect.

CONSTITUENTS
- 1 part Skullcap (*Scutellaria lateriflora*)
- 1 part Valerian (*Valeriana officinalis*)

FORM

Capsule.

DOSAGE

One "00" capsule with meals. Taken at bedtime for insomnia.

INDICATION

Nervousness, nervous stomach, insomnia, restlessness, fidgetiness, mouth and throat dry. The tongue tends to be dry and red or dark red, while the pulse tends to be deep, thready and rapid. Nerve rings tend to be present in the iris.

APPLICATION

Insomnia, neurasthenia, restlessness, stress-induced indigestion.

CONTRAINDICATION

Contraindicated for a person who gets groggy from Valerian.

HERBS AND ACTIONS

Skullcap is a central nervous system calmative with indirect effects on the gastrointestinal tract. Valerian is a central nervous system calmative with direct tonic effects on the digestive system.

MODIFICATION

For insomnia of longer duration, add Avena and Lemon Balm.

COMMENTARY

This is one of Dr. Carroll's most popular formulas for calming the nerves. It has a wide range of use and can be used for many purposes from insomnia to indigestion. This is a classic example of a naturopathic herbal formula, where an action is directed at the nervous system, but the end result affects the digestive system, upon which a bulk of our health is dependent.

Nerve Remedy

Therapeutic Principle
Sedative.

Constituents
- 1 ounce Cypripedium (*Cypripedium pubescens*)
- ½ ounce Chamomile (*Anthemis nobilis*)

Form
Tincture.

Dosage
Fifteen to thirty drops, depending on the seriousness of the condition.

Indication
Insomnia, fidgetiness, excessive dreaming. The tongue is usually red and the pulse usually wiry. Nerve rings can be present in the iris.

Application
Insomnia, neurasthenia.

Contraindication
Contraindicated in pregnancy.

Herbs and Actions
Cypripedium acts as a relaxant, nervine, parodyne, anti-spasmodic and mild tonic. Chamomile acts as a relaxant, tonic, and anti-spasmodic.

Modifications
For a stronger sedative effect, add Valerian and Skullcap. For a more tonifying effect, add Mother's Wort.

COMMENTARY
This remedy comes out of the Thomsonian and Physio-Medicalist schools. It appears in Clymer's (1902) book **Medicines of Nature**.

The roots of Cypripedium were introduced to medical practice by Dr. Samuel Thomson. Dr. Cook said about the roots of Cypripedium:

"They are nearly pure relaxants, with not enough stimulation to be available. Their influence is manifested slowly, and is expended wholly upon the nervous system; and it is only through the nervous tissues that they impress other parts....They are used in all the multiplied forms of nervous irritability and excitement, except when arising from advancing putrescence. They soothe and calm the entire system, easing all forms of pain growing out of local or general irritation, and inducing quiet and usually securing sleep (Cook, 1869)."

Dr. Nowell's General Nervine Tonic

THERAPEUTIC PRINCIPLE
Sedative.

CONSTITUENTS
- 1 part Skullcap Powder (*Scutellaria lateriflora*)
- 1 part Hops Powder (*Humulus lupulus*)
- 1 part Valerian root Powder (*Valerian officinalis*)
- 1 part Gum Asafoetida Powder (*Ferula foetida*)
- 1 part Gentian Root (*Gentiana lutea*)

FORM
Capsule.

DOSAGE
Take one to two capsules three times per day.

INDICATION
Nervousness, insomnia, fidgeting, excessive dreams, palpitations. The tongue tends to be red and the pulse wiry. Nerve rings can be present in the iris.

Application
Insomnia, neurasthenia.

Contraindication
Contraindicated in pregnancy.

Herbs and Actions
Skullcap acts as a sedative, tonic, and anti-spasmodic. Hops acts as a hypnotic, sedative, and tonic. Hops and valerian work as a pair for anti-spasmodic properties for coughs and nervous spasmodic conditions. Valerian acts as an anti-spasmodic, calmative, hypnotic, and nervine. Asafoetida acts as an anti-spasmodic and sedative. Gentian acts as a tonic and stomachic, strengthening the activity of the stomach and improving digestion.

Modifications
With palpitations, add Hawthorne. With more fidgeting and insomnia, add Passion Flower and Chamomile. With nervous stomach, add Chamomile.

Commentary
This formula was used by Dr. Nowell, the founder of the Dominion Herbal College. It contains the small formula of Skullcap, Hops, and Valerian within it. These have stood the test of time as general nervines. The addition of Gentian as a digestive tonic and stomachic leads to improving the general vitality of the patient and strengthening and tonifying the nervous system by improving digestion.

Weiss' Nerve Tea

Therapeutic Principle
Sedative.

Constituents
- 2 parts Angelica Root (*Angelica archangelica*)
- 1 part Rosemary Leaf (*Rosmarinus officinalis*)
- 3 parts Melissa Leaf (*Melissa officinalis*)
- 1 part Lavender Flower (*Lavendula officinalis*)
- 2 parts Hops Leaf (*Humulus lupulus*)
- 1 part Yarrow Herb (*Achillea millefolium*)

Form
Infusion.

Dosage
One cup three times per day.

Indication
Insomnia, nervousness, excessive dreaming. The tongue is usually red and the pulse is usually wiry. Nerve rings can be present in the iris.

Application
Insomnia, restlessness.

Contraindication
Contraindicated in pregnancy.

Herbs and Actions
The herbs act synergistically as a calming sedative. Angelica acts as a nervine and tonic. Rosemary acts as an anti-spasmodic. Melissa acts as a calmative and nervine, anti-spasmotic and relaxant. Lavender acts as a sedative and anti-spasmodic. Hops acts as an anodyne, hypnotic, sedative, and tonic. Yarrow acts as an anti-spasmodic and tonic.

Modification

For mild functional depression, add Hypericum.

Commentary

This formula was recorded by Rudolf Fritz Weiss in ***Herbal Medicine*** (1988). He was a medical doctor and one of the leading medical herbalists in Germany. His book has been a standard text in Naturopathic medical schools for years. This formula combines hypnotics, sedatives, nervines, calmatives, and anti-spasmodics with herbs that are tonifying and nutritive to the nervous system.

16

The Resuscitating Formulas

Use

- To restore consciousness and alertness.
- To tonify the nervous system.

Formulas

Cook's Restorative Compound

THERAPEUTIC PRINCIPLE

Resuscitating formula.

CONSTITUENTS

- 3 ounces Lavender flowers (*Lavendula officinalis*)
- 1 ounce Cinnamon (*Cinnamomum zeylanicum*)
- 1 ounce Ginger (*Zingiber officinale*)
- 1 ounce Mace (*Myristica moschata*)
- 1 ounce Anise (*Pimpinella anisum*)
- 1 ounce Mother's Wort (*Leonurus cardiaca*)

FORM

Compounded tincture. Percolate the herbs with one pint of brandy, then with diluted alcohol until a quart is obtained (Cook,1869; Bergner,1999).

Dosage

30 drops under the tongue. Half a fluid drachm or more, as required.

Indication

Weakness, fainting. The pulse is usually weak and the tongue quivering.

Application

Faintness, fainting, sympathetic palpitation, colic.

Contraindication

Contraindicated in pregnancy.

Herbs and Actions

The herbs act to awaken the vital energy of the body. All of the aromatic herbs open the orifices of the head. These are stimulating herbs. Lavender acts as a stimulant, influencing the nervous peripheries, and is indicated in prostration.

Modification

If the body is cold, add drop dosages of Aconite. By adding Rosemary, Cloves, and Red Saunders and removing Ginger, Anise, and Mother's Wort, we have compound spirits of Lavender.

Commentary

This formula is from the nineteenth century Physio-Medical system. The Physio-Medical system was a medical herbalism system that evolved out of Thomsonian herbalism. It was recorded by Dr. William Cook, professor of botany, therapeutics, and material medica in the Physio-Medical Institute, in the ***Physio-Medical Dispensatory*** in 1869. It contains a wealth of knowledge about the medical uses of herbs.

Shock and Collapse Formula

Therapeutic Principle
Resuscitating formula.

Constituents
- 1 part Myrrh (*Commiphora myrrha*)
- ¼ part Cayenne (*Capsicum minimum*)
- 2 parts Echinacea (*Echinachea angustifolia*)

Form
Tincture.

Dosage
10 to 15 drops in plenty of water.

Indication
Collapse, fainting, shock. The pulse is usually weak.

Application
Shock, collapse, prostration, profound congestions, externally for rheumatism, neuralgia, sprains, bruises, fresh cuts, or indolent ulcers, to prevent mortification (Christopher, 1976).

Contraindication
Contraindicated in pregnancy.

Herbs and Actions

Myrrh acts as a stimulant and a stimulating tonic. It increases the fullness and force of the pulse, and exerts a well-marked influence on the capillary circulation (Cook, 1869). Cayenne acts as an intense stimulant, a circulatory stimulant, and a nervous system stimulant. It increases the power of each pulse. Echinacea restores capillary circulation and stimulates the functional activity of the kidneys, all of the glandular organs, the lymphatic system, the stomach, and the bowels (Ellingwood, 1919).

Modification

If extremities are cold, add drop doses of Aconite.

Commentary

Cayenne by itself can resuscitate. It was a major stimulant used by Dr. Samuel Thomson and Dr. Cook said that cayenne is "one of the purest of all known stimulants, of great intensity, very permanent in its action, spreading through the entire system rather slowly, but ultimately reaching every organ of the frame (Cook, 1869)." Cook goes on to say that Cayenne:

"....first shows its power upon the heart and the large and central blood vessels; but finally transverses from the center to the very capillaries. It thus slowly gives increased tone to the circulation – not so materially increasing the frequency of the pulse, as giving power to each pulsation. In cases where the pulse is enfeebled and very much hurried from putrescent tendencies, as in typhus, malignant scarlatina, phlegmonous erysipelas, gangrenous wounds, threatened absorption of pus, etc., capsicum may be used in full quantities, and will be followed by diminished frequency but greater firmness of the arterial action...In the collapsed stage of cholera, of yellow fever, of all clammy sweats; also in asthmatic asphyxia and collapse from burns or other profound shock of injury, it is one of the best agents to secure full reactions (Cook, 1865)."

The Astringent Formulas

Use

- Contain tannins, organic acids, and inorganic salts.
- To stop bleeding.
- To regulate the smooth muscles of the genitourinary tract, gastrointestinal tract, respiratory tract, and blood vessels.
- For cough, bleeding, diarrhea, leukorrhea, spermatorrhea, excess urine or sweat.

Formulas

Diarrhea Powders

THERAPEUTIC PRINCIPLE
Anti-diarrhetic.

Constituents

- 4 ounces Bayberry (*Myrica cerifera*)
- 4 ounces Goldenseal (*Hydrastis canadensis*)
- 4 ounces Rhubarb (*Rheum palmatum*)
- 1 ounce Saleratus (*Celatrus scandens*)
- ½ ounce Myrrh (*Commiphora myrrha*)
- 2 ounces Cinnamon (*Cinnamomum zeylanicum*)
- 2 ounces Peppermint (*Mentha piperita*)
- 1 pound sugar

Form

Powder.

Dosage

One teaspoon three times per day.

Indication

Diarrhea, loss of appetite, indigestion, abdominal pain, tenesmus, malaise. The tongue tends to be pale or with a white coating. The pulse can be slow.

Application

Diarrhea, dysentery, colitis.

Contraindication

Contraindicated in pregnancy.

Herbs and Actions

The herbs act synergistically to stop diarrhea. Bayberry acts as an astringent and anti-diarrhetic. Goldenseal is a tonic with specific action on gastrointestinal mucus membranes and anti-diarrhetic. Rhubarb acts as an astringent and anti-diarrhetic. It is a tonic to the duodenum and small intestines. Myrrh acts as an astringent and tonic, combined with bayberry. It can stop passive hemorrhage of the bowels. Cinnamon is warming and an astringent. It is indicated in looseness of the bowels with gripping and flatulence. Peppermint acts as an anti-spasmodic and carminative. It acts as an adjuvant in preparations for diarrhea.

Modifications
Blackberry Root can be added for stubborn cases of diarrhea.

Commentary
This is a Thomsonian formula, originally from Dr. Samuel Thomson, probably the most influential herbalist in American history.

Sumach Astringent

Therapeutic Principle
Formula for leukorrhea.

Constituents
- 1 part Sumach Berries (*Rhus glabra*)
- 1 part Sumach Bark (*Rhus glabra*)
- 1 part White Pine Bark (*Pinus strobus*)
- 1 part Slippery Elm Bark (*Ulmus fulva*)

Form
Decoction.

Dosage
One cup three times per day.

Indication
Leukorrhea, pale face, malaise, loose stool. The tongue tends to be pale and the pulse weak and soft.

Application
Leukorrhea.

Contraindication
None known.

Herbs and Actions

Sumach acts as an astringent and tonic, stopping leukorrhea. White Pine acts as a demulcent and diuretic, having a tonifying effect upon the bladder and kidneys. Slippery elm acts as a demulcent, especially good for mucus irritations.

Modifications

With abdominal pain add Fennel and Orange Peel.

Commentary

This formula is recorded by Dr. Christopher. These are all herbs that Samuel Thomson used in his medical system. Sumach was one of Dr. Thomson's favorite herbs, having borrowed it from the American Indians. He used it quite often with children and especially with canker sores. Cankers were obstructions to health that attached themselves to mucus membranes, causing disease and putrefaction.

Ellingwood's Hemostatic

Therapeutic Principle

Hemostatic and anti-hemorrhage.

Constituents

- Cinnamon Bark Oil (*Cinnamomum zeylanicum*)
- Erigeron Flower oil (*Erigeron canadensis*)

Form

Tincture.

Dosage

Ten to thirty drops on sugar, or dropped at once on water, will control nearly every controllable passive hemorrhage.

Indication

Hemorrhage, uterine hemorrhage, menorrhagia, abdominal pain, bleeding after abortion, delivery, or during pregnancy, pulmonary hemorrhage, persistent hemoptysis, gastric and intestinal hemorrhages, hematuria, and nasal hemorrhage.

Application

Threatened abortion, menorrhagia, uterine bleeding, vaginal bleeding during pregnancy or after childbirth, tuberculosis, ulcerative colitis, epistaxis, hemoptysis, hematemesis, spitting and coughing with blood.

Herbs and Actions

Cinnamon acts as an astringent and hemostatic and acts in perfect harmony with Erigeron for all passive hemorrhages. Erigeron acts as an astringent, hemostatic, and diffusive stimulant.

Modifications

If bleeding is excessive, add Agrimony. With bleeding from mucus membranes, add Goldenseal. With coldness in the extremities, add Composition powder. Can be combined with turpentine to improve hemostatic effectiveness.

Commentary

This formula was developed by one of the great eclectic physicians, Dr. Finley Ellingwood. He used the formula as his first resort in passive hemorrhages. The formula can irritate the stomach, especially if used over a period of time.

18

The Anti-parasitic Formulas

Use

- For parasitic infestations.
- For chronic abdominal pain.
- For chronic diarrhea.

Formulas

Ring's Entozoic

THERAPEUTIC PRINCIPLE
Anti-parasitic.

CONSTITUENTS
- 1 part Pinkroot (*Spigelia marilandica*)
- 1 part Swamp Milkweed (*Asclepias incarnata*)
- 1 part Mayapple (*Podophyllum peltatum*)
- 1 part Bitterroot (*Apocynum cannabinum*)
- 2 parts Balmony (*Chelone glabra*)

FORM
Tincture.

Dosage
15 drops.

Indication
Recurrent abdominal pain, vomiting, chronic diarrhea. The tongue can be geographic.

Application
Ascariasis, parasitic infestations, biliary ascariasis, chronic dysentery, chronic gastritis.

Contraindication
Contraindicated in pregnancy. This formula contains toxic botanicals and should be administered by skilled professionals only.

Herbs and Actions
Pinkroot is specific in the removal of intestinal worms. Swamp Milkweed is an anthelmintic and stomachic. Mayapple acts as an alterative and liver stimulant. Bitterroot is a circulatory stimulant. Balmony is a vermifuge but is chiefly used to give tone to the digestive system that should accompany and follow anthelmintics.

Modifications
To increase the anthelmintic effect, add Wormwood. To excrete the parasite through the stool, add Rhubarb. If hands and feet are cold, add Cinnamon and Ginger. This should be followed by a purging dose of Epsom salts or Senna.

Commentary
This is an anti-parasite formula from one of the great physicians from the Eclectic school of Therapeutic Herbalism. It is most safely taken followed by a purging dose of Epsom salts (Boyle, 1993). Eclecticism was an herbal medical sect founded by A. Wooster Beach.

Worm Syrup

Therapeutic Principle
Anti-parasitic.

Constituents
- 4 ounce Butternut Bark (*Juglans cinera*)
- 2 ounce Sage (*Salvia officinalis*)
- 2 ounce Myrrh (*Commiphora myrrha*)
- 2 ounce Poplar Bark (*Populus tremuloides*)
- 4 ounce Bitterroot (*Apocynum cannabinum*)

Form
Syrup.

Dosage
One teaspoonful three times per day.

Indication
Recurrent abdominal pain, vomiting, chronic diarrhea. The tongue can be geographic.

Application
Ascariasis, parasitic infestations, ringworm, biliary ascariasis, chronic dysentery, chronic gastritis.

Herbs and Actions
Butternut acts as an anthelmintic, cathartic, stimulant and influences the liver and gall bladder. Sage acts as a tonic, relaxant and mild stimulant. Myrrh acts as an antiseptic, stimulating tonic and induces gastric excitement. Poplar acts as an anthelmintic and tonic. Bitterroot is a circulatory stimulant.

Modifications

To increase the anti-parasitic effect, add Black Walnut. Add Uva Ursi with catarrh of the bladder. This should be followed by a dose of Senna.

Commentary

This is a Thomsonian formula also recorded by Benjamin Colby (1846). Samuel Thomson created an entire system of medicine that greatly influenced this country. He patented a system, "Thomson's Improved System of Botanic Practice of Medicine," that he would sell "Family Rights" to people to use.

Vermifuge Formula

Therapeutic Principle

Anti-parasitic.

Constituents

- ½ ounce Tansy herb (*Tanacetum vulgare*)
- ½ ounce Wormwood herb (*Artemesia absinthium*)
- ½ ounce Santonica buds (*Artemesia santonica*)
- ½ ounce Chamomile flowers (*Matricaria chamomilla*)

Form

Decoction.

Dosage

One-half cup three times per day.

Indication

Recurrent abdominal pain, vomiting, chronic diarrhea, the tongue can be geographic.

Application

Parasitic infestation, ascariasis, biliary ascariasis, chronic dysentery, chronic gastritis.

Contraindication
Contraindicated in pregnancy.

Herbs and Actions
Tansy acts as an anthelmintic and tonic. Wormwood is used as an anthelmintic and to tonify a flaccid abdomen. Santonica is a vermifuge, working against round, tape, and pin worms. Chamomile acts as an antispasmodic, aromatic, bitter tonic, and stimulant stomachic.

Modifications
Can be followed by a dose of Senna to purge and help remove parasites. If hands and feet are cold, add Cinnamon and Ginger.

Commentary
This old formula was used by Potter, Dr. Shook, and Dr. Christopher. It is a classic example of having an herb added to assist in the primary function of the formula. The Tansy, Wormwood, and Santonica are all anthelmintic in action. The Chamomile acts as an anti-spasmodic, aromatic, bitter tonic, and stimulant stomachic. Chamomile helps balance and soothe the anthelmintic actions of the other herbs. It can help with flatulent colic, dyspepsia, spasms, stomach cramps, and is good for fever and restlessness in children.

Young Deer's Formula for Infantile Worms

Therapeutic Principle
Anti-parasitic.

Constituents
- Sassafras (*Sassafras albidum*)
- Dogwood (*Cornus florida*)
- Service Tree (*Amelanchier arborea*)
- Black Gum (*Nyssa sylvatica*)
- Wild Rose Root, both small and large spp. (*Rosa lucida*)

Form
Decoction.

Dosage
The doctor takes the decoction in his or her mouth and then blows it upon the head and hands of the patient. The child drinks a little of the medicine at the end of each treatment.

Indication
Infant with nervousness and troubled sleep, child wakes suddenly crying as if frightened, dark circles under the eyes of an adult.

Application
Parasites, worms.

Herbs and Actions
Sassafras is used as a vermifuge and to purify the blood. Dogwood is used as a vermifuge and tonic. Service Tree is used as a vermifuge and tonic. Black Gum is used as a vermifuge. Wild Rose is used as a vermifuge.

Modifications
Can be combined with Sweetgum for nervousness.

Commentary
This formula is recorded by James Mooney in ***Sacred Formulas of the Cherokee*** (1891). He obtained the formula from Young Deer, and it is used for a disease called Gunwanigistai, or "something is causing something to eat or gnaw the vitals of the patient." The herbal formula is always given with a verbal formula, or prayer. There are specific instructions for the preparation of this herbal formula:

"The bark in every case is taken from the east side of the tree, and the roots selected are also generally, if not always, those growing toward the east. In this case the roots and barks are not bruised, but are simply steeped in warm water for four days. The child is then stripped and bathed all over with the decoction morning and night for four days, no formula being used during the bathing. It is then made to hold up its hands in front of its face with the palms turned out toward the doctor, who takes some of the medicine in his mouth and repeats the prayer mentally, blowing the medicine upon the head and hands of the patient at the final '*Yu!*' of each paragraph....The child drinks a little medicine at the end of each treatment (Mooney, 1891)."

19

The Purgative Formulas

Use

- To purge and cleanse the gastrointestinal tract.
- To remove toxins from the gastrointestinal tract.
- To cleanse and detoxify the body for bio-purification.
- To remove parasites.

Formulas

42 Capsules

Therapeutic Principle

Purgative; laxative with a cold nature.

Constituents

- 2 parts Wormwood (*Artemsia absinthium*)
- 1 part Cape Aloes (*Aloes socotrina*)

Form

Capsules, "00" size.

Dosage

One "00" capsule per day acts as a strong laxative. In more difficult cases, two capsules may be taken every four hours until there is bowel movement. A "42" Cocktail consists of two "42" Capsules emptied into a glass, mixed with one ounce of warm water, and drunk. This is followed by a chaser of more warm water to clean the herbs out of the glass and wash the bitter taste away. The next meal should be skipped (Boyle, 1988).

Indications

Excessive symptoms in the bowels, such as constipation, fever, abdominal fullness, delirium, irritability, tongue yellow and prickly, pulse deep and forceful. There can also be dryness in the intestines with abdominal pain, and a dry mouth and tongue. Watch for signs and symptoms of the beginning of a cold, or a cold in progress, acute conditions, pain, dizziness and seizures.

Application

Constipation, atonic dyspepsia, round worms, pinworms, colds, angina, asthma, acute conditions with pain and irritation, acute appendicitis, acute cholecystitis, syncope, seizures.

Contraindications

Contraindications are nausea (unless due to food poisoning), intestinal obstruction.

Herbs and Actions

The Wormwood acts on the upper gastrointestinal tract while the Cape Aloes is a slow large intestine purgative which empties the bowel in 10-15 hours.

Modifications

Add one part Gentian (*Gentiana lutea*) to make a combination digestive aid and laxative. This makes Dr. Carroll's "C" Capsules, with the Gentian stimulating HCl. Dosage is one capsule per day in warm water.

Commentary

This is a formula from Dr. O.G. Carroll, an influential naturopath from the early part of this century. It is a standard of treatment in many naturopathic circles, used for most anything as a beginning point within the tenants of nature cure. It is used extensively at the naturopathic school clinics and by those influenced by Dr. Harold Dick. The "42" Cocktail is indicated in acute conditions with pain and irritation. Colds may be aborted if a "42" Cocktail is taken and the next two meals are skipped.

Dr. Carroll's "C" Capsules

Therapeutic Principle

Laxative with a cold nature.

Constituents

- 2 parts Wormwood (*Artemesia absinthium*)
- 1 part Gentian (*Gentiana lutea*)
- 1 part Cape Aloes (*Aloes socotrina*)

Form

Capsules.

Dosage

One "00" capsule per day in warm water.

Indication

For indigestion and food stagnation with symptoms such as fullness and distension in the gastric region, belching, acid regurgitation, loss of appetite, constipation, abdominal pain. The tongue may be yellow and dry, while the pulse can by deep and slippery.

Application

Constipation, indigestion, abdominal pain, food stagnation, loss of appetite.

Contraindication
Contraindicated in pregnancy and deficiency states.

Herbs and Actions
The Wormwood is tonic to the upper gastrointestinal tract. The Gentian stimulates the production of hydrochloric acid. The powdered gum of Cape Aloe is tonic to the lower gastrointestinal tract. The Wormwood and Cape Aloe together act as a downward bearing purgative.

Modification
Remove the Gentian and it acts as a stronger purgative. This is Dr. Carroll's "42" Capsules. Add Skullcap if indigestion is due to stress and nervousness and there is much flatulence.

Commentary
This is a commonly used capsule developed by Dr. O.G. Carroll (1879-1962), a turn-of-the-century naturopath and the founder of constitutional hydrotherapy. His herbalism was strongly influenced by Father Kneipp and Samuel Thompson. The design of this formula is a classic example of the modification of an existing formula to change its intensity of action and trophism. It is the addition of Gentian to the "42"Capsules, with the dosage decreased. This changes the focus from more of a purgative laxative to also focusing on indigestion.

Intestinal Broom

Therapeutic Principle
Laxative, mild purgative

Constituents

- 6 parts Ground Senna Leaves (*Cassia marilandica*)
- 3 parts Ground Buckthorn Bark (*Rhamnus frangula*)
- 1 part Ground Psyllium Seed Husks (*Plantago psyllium*)
- 1/10th part Powdered Sassafras Root Bark (*Sassafras albidum*)
- ½ part Ground Dark Anise Seed (*Pimpinella anisum*)
- 1/10th part Ground Buchu Leaves (*Barosma betulina*)
- ½ part Ground Blonde Psyllium Seed (*Plantago psyllium*)
- 1/8th part Powdered Irish Moss (*Chondrus crispus*)
- 1/8th part Granulated Agar-Agar (*Gelidium amansii*)
- 1/2th part Ground Dark Fennel Seed (*Foeniculum vulgare*)

Form

Powder

Dosage

One-half teaspoon with a glass of water. Can also be sprinkled over salads or brewed as a tea.

Indication

Constipation, irregular bowels, toxemia, polysystemic candadiasis, cold.

Application

Constipation, detoxification, cancer prevention.

Herbs and Actions

Senna acts as a laxative and cathartic. Buckthorn acts as a laxative and purgative. Psyllium acts as a laxative. Sassafras acts as an alterative. Anise acts as a tonic, antispasmodic, carminative, digestive, and stomachic. Buchu acts as a carminative, diuretic, and stimulant. Irish Moss acts as a demulcent and is mucilaginous. Agar-agar acts as a laxative, absorbing and retaining moisture. Fennel acts as a carminative, antispasmodic, diuretic, stimulant, and stomachic.

MODIFICATIONS

Fresh ground Flax Seed can be added for more lubrication to the large intestine. Bentonite clay can be added for more absorption. Rhubarb root can be added to relieve pain.

COMMENTARY

This formula is from Professor Arnold Ehret. He wrote ***Mucusless Diet Healing System***, and his dietary regimens influenced many people, including Dr. Benedict Lust, the founder of Naturopathy. Benedict Lust learned his herbalism from Father Sebastian Kneipp, one of the most famous nature doctors of all time. This formula has influenced many modern fiber formulas, serving as the basis for the design of a well-rounded herbal formula to cleanse the intestines. It was recorded by John Lust, the nephew of Benedict Lust, in ***The Herb Book*** (1974), one of the best small handbooks on herbal medicine.

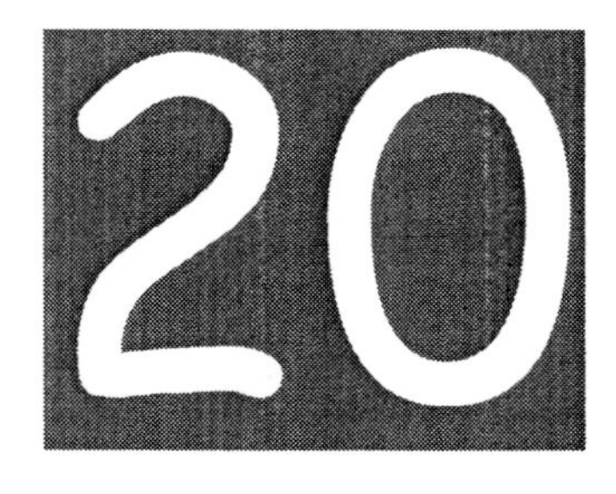

The Emetic Formulas

Use

- To induce emesis.
- To cleanse and detoxify the upper gastrointestinal tract.
- To cleanse and detoxify the upper respiratory tract.
- To prevent asthma.

Formulas

Emetic Powder

THERAPEUTIC PRINCIPLE
Emetic.

CONSTITUENTS
- 4 ounce Lobelia herb (*Lobelia inflata*)
- 4 ounce Lobelia seed (*Lobelia inflata*)
- 2 ounce Bayberry (*Myrica cerifera*)
- 4 ounce Cayenne (*Capsicum frutescens*)
- 2 ounce Valerian (*Valeriana officinalis*)

FORM
Powder.

Dosage
Drink one cup of tea until emesis occurs.

Indication
Digestion upset, excess phlegm, indigestion, food poisoning, fullness. The pulse tends to be slippery and the tongue usually has a thick coating.

Application
Indigestion, food poisoning, acute jaundice, acute infection, mushroom poisoning, liver disease.

Contraindications
Contraindicated in pregnancy.

Herbs and Actions
Lobelia acts as an emetic, relaxant, and sialagogue. Cayenne acts as a stimulant and excites the stomach. Bayberry works as a pair with Lobelia, being a stimulant and astringent, and causing contractions and stimulation of the stomach. Valerian acts as a nervine and relaxant, calming the action of the emetic after the process is complete.

Modifications
Follow emetic with tonifying herbs, to gently restore the system, such as Nettles, Raspberry, or Chamomile. With fever and lung problem, follow with Mullein and Coltsfoot.

Commentary
This is a Thomsonian formula. Samuel Thomson developed a patented system of medicine based around Lobelia and its actions. Thomsonian herbalism combined herbs used by the Europeans and the American Indians into a cohesive system. They also applied hydrotherapy and were known to "sweat and puke" their patients. Samuel Thomson would follow emesis with an enema to unload the bowels, and after a rest of one to two hours, would follow with a steam or tepid sponge bath.

Cook's Emetic Course of Medicine

Therapeutic Principle
Emetic.

Constituents
- First Course: Two drams of powdered Lobelia herb (*Lobelia inflata*)
- Second Course: Two ounces Composition Powder drink
- Third Course: Cayenne (*Capsicum frutescens*)
- Fourth Course: 2 parts Ginger (*Zingiber officinale*)
  2 parts Geranium (*Geranium maculatum*)
  6 parts Swamp Milkweed (*Asclepias incarnata*)
- Fifth Course: Lobelia injection of Bowels

Form
A sequenced course of herbs.

Dosage
Follow each course.

Indication
Digestive upset, chills, spasms, fever, acute disease, excessive mucus, cholecystitis, dyspepsia, indigestion, hyperacidity, diarrhea. The pulse tends to be slippery and the tongue usually has a thick coating.

Application
Necessary evacuation of contents of stomach, colic, cholera, recurrent fever, excessive mucus, asthma, hypochlorydia, dyspepsia, dysentery, diarrhea, chronic liver disease.

Contraindication
Contraindicated in pregnancy.

Herbs and Actions

Capsicum acts as a stimulant and excites the stomach. Ginger is a stimulant, aromatic, a sialagogue, and increases the flow of mucus from the lungs. Geranium is a stimulant with tonic properties. Asclepias provokes emesis and is a relaxant. Lobelia acts as a relaxant, sialagogue and emetic.

Modification

With liver disease, follow with Milk Thistle, Taraxacum. With fever, follow with Peppermint, Yarrow.

Commentary

This course of herbs for emesis was discussed by William Cook, MD, in the Physio-Medical Dispensatory. Dr. Cook was professor of botany, therapeutics, and material media in the Physio-Medical Institute and professor of surgery in the Physio-Medical College of Ohio. He claims that this course of medicine was actually discovered by Samuel Thomson, and that this discovery "would have deserved the highest honors due a benefactor and a man of genius, had he never performed any other labor for his race (Cook, 1869)." Cook summed up the use of emetics under the general rule:

"Give them when the stomach and liver are oppressed with unhealthy secretions and morbific materials, which are not likely to be removed in safe season by other measures; and when accumulation in these organs are not only weighing upon other portions of the frame, but when they are oppressing the nervous system and are proving decided obstacles in the way of an equalized circulation (Cook, 1869)." He felt that "in febrile cases, suitable diaphoretics are to follow an emetic; while in all chronic cases, proper tonics and cathartics (usually hepatics) are required (Cook, 1869)."

The Obstetrical Formulas

Use

- With childbirth.
- For conception.

Formulas

Mother's Cordial

Therapeutic Principle
Tonify the uterus.

Constituents
- 1 pound Partridge Berry (*Mitchella repens*)
- 4 ounces False Unicorn Root (*Chamaelirium luteum*)
- 4 ounces Blue Cohosh (*Caulophyllum thalictroides*)
- 4 ounces Cramp Bark (*Viburnum opulus*)

Form
Tincture.

Dosage
One large tablespoon three to four times per day or more.

INDICATION
Uterine problems, nervous disorders, weakness of the back, leukorrhea, prolapse, cramps, failure to conceive, persistent menstruation, laxity of pelvic organs.

APPLICATION
Uterine laxity, uterine tonic, leukorrhea, prolapse, infertility, menorrhagia.

CONTRAINDICATIONS
Contraindicated in first two trimesters of pregnancy.

HERBS AND ACTIONS
Partridge Berry acts as a uterine tonic and is anti-spasmodic to the uterus. False Unicorn Root acts as a uterine tonic and nutritive. Blue Cohosh acts as a parturient and anti-spasmodic. It is tonic to the female reproductive system. Cramp Bark acts as a uterine anti-spasmodic with gentle tonic properties.

MODIFICATIONS
Combine one ounce of Celastrus with one pint of Mother's cordial to treat spermatorrhea.

COMMENTARY
This formula was introduced by Dr. Sweet, a Thomsonian physician from Connecticut, in 1826. He published the formula in the Botanic Vindicator and other journals, and it was used by the Thomsonian herbalists, the Eclectics, the Physio-Medicalists, and today's modern Naturopaths and Medical Herbalists. Dr. Cook (1869) "felt that few compounds in the whole range of Pharmacy are so mild in action, yet at the same time so reliable." Cook describes the unique process to make this compound:

"Crush well, and macerate for three days in a sufficient quantity of diluted alcohol. Transfer to a percolator, treat with diluted alcohol, and reserve the first three pints that pass; then treat with boiling water till exhausted, add two pounds of sugar, evaporate to two pints, and mix with the reserved liquid. Some speak of using brandy instead of diluted alcohol… (Cook, 1869)."

Ellingwood's Hemostatic

Therapeutic Principle

Hemostatic and anti-hemorrhage.

Constituents

- Cinnamon Bark Oil (*Cinnamomum zeylanicum*)
- Erigeron Flower oil (*Erigeron canadensis*)

Form

Tincture.

Dosage

Ten to thirty drops on sugar, or dropped at once on water, will control nearly every controllable passive hemorrhage.

Indication

Hemorrhage, uterine hemorrhage, menorrhagia, abdominal pain, bleeding after abortion, delivery, or during pregnancy, pulmonary hemorrhage, persistent hemoptysis, gastric and intestinal hemorrhages, hematuria, and nasal hemorrhage.

Application

Threatened abortion, menorrhagia, uterine bleeding, vaginal bleeding during pregnancy or after childbirth, tuberculosis, ulcerative colitis, epistaxis, hemoptysis, hematemesis, spitting and coughing with blood.

Herbs and Actions

Cinnamon acts as an astringent and hemostatic and acts in perfect harmony with Erigeron for all passive hemorrhages. Erigeron acts as an astringent, hemostatic, and diffusive stimulant.

Modifications

If bleeding is excessive, add Agrimony. With bleeding from mucus membranes, add Goldenseal. With coldness in the extremities, add Composition powder. Can be combined with turpentine to improve hemostatic effectiveness.

COMMENTARY

Dr. Ellingwood wrote ***American Materia Medica, Therapeutics and Pharmacognosy,*** a large volume on eclectic medical herbalism. He felt that the formula "works to a better advantage in hemorrhage due to atonic conditions of the non-gravid womb, or where there is muscular relaxation, or a general flaccid state of the womb after delivery....It certainly restores tone to the uterine muscular structure and induces tonic contraction. In some cases, during labor, it promotes the normal labor pains and materially increases uterine contraction, and prevents postpartum hemorrhage. Midwives and old nurses have long given a strong infusion of cinnamon to control postpartum hemorrhage, and it has been advised in "nose bleed" and in flooding during miscarriage and in menorrhagia."

Anti-Miscarriage Formula

THERAPEUTIC PRINCIPLE

Anti-abortifacient.

CONSTITUENTS

- False Unicorn (*Chamaelirium luteum*)
- Lobelia (*Lobelia inflata*)

FORM

Tea.

DOSAGE

One Teaspoon of herbs to a cup of water.

INDICATIONS

Pregnancy with spotting, hemorrhaging, weakened conditions of the reproductive organs.

APPLICATION

Threatened abortion, pregnancy with spotting, hemorrhaging.

CONTRAINDICATION

See a physician with these indications.

Herbs and Actions

False Unicorn Root tonifies female reproductive organs, improving their function and nutrition. Lobelia acts as a relaxant.

Commentary

This is a formula recorded by Dr. Christopher. He is using Thomsonian herbalism in a very simple formula. He said that if hemorrhaging starts, "...stay in bed, use a pan when needed, and use ½ cup of this tea each ½ hour until bleeding stops, then each waking hour for one day, while in bed as much as possible, then three times in a day for three weeks (Christopher, 1976)."

22

The Cancer Formulas

Use

- To treat and prevent cancer.
- To eliminate toxins and abscesses.
- To increase blood circulation and lymphatic circulation.
- To eliminate tumors and masses.
- For tonification.

Formulas

Eli Jones' Syrup/Compound Syrup Scrophularia

THERAPEUTIC PRINCIPLE

Alterative, lymphatic and glandular alterative, anti-cancer.

Constituents

- 32 ounces Figwort (*Scrophularia nodosa*)
- 8 ounces Poke Root (*Phytolacca americana*)
- 8 ounces Yellow Dock (*Rumex crispus*)
- 4 ounces False Bittersweet (*Celastrus scandens*)
- 2 ounces Corydalis (*Corydalis formosa*)
- 4 ounces Mayapple (*Podophyllum peltatum*)
- 3 ounces Juniper Berries (*Juniperis communis*)
- 1 ounce Prickly Ash (*Zanthoxylum spp.*)
- 2 ounces Guaiacum Wood (*Guaiacum officinale*)
- Oil of Sassafras (*Sassafras albidum*)

Form

Syrup.

Dosage

One tablespoon three times per day or enough to keep the bowels regular.

Indication

Tumors, fixed pain, glandular swelling, constipation. The pulse tends to be wiry. The tongue can be dark red. The lymphatic rosary can be present in the iris.

Application

Tumors, cancer, liver congestion, lymphatic congestion, constipation, detoxification, skin disorders.

Contraindications

Contraindicated in pregnancy and nursing mothers.

Herbs and Actions

Figwort acts as an alterative with particular affinity to the glandular system and the blood. Pokeroot acts as an alterative and lymphagogue. Yellow Dock acts as an alterative, tonic, and blood purifier. False Bittersweet acts as an alterative. Corydalis acts as an alterative, tonic, anodyne, anti-cancer, and detoxicant. Mayapple acts as a purgative, alterative, and anti-cancer. Juniper Berries tonify the kidneys and assist in elimination of waste. Prickly ash acts as an alterative, particularly acting upon glands, the kidney, bladder, and spleen. Guaiacum acts as a laxative and stimulant, increasing vital heat and circulation. Sassafras acts as an alterative.

Modifications

Remove Sassafras, Guaiacum, Prickly Ash, Juniper, False Bittersweet, and Poke Root to form Scudder's Alterative.

Commentary

This formula was made famous as a cancer remedy by Eli Jones, MD. He wrote a monumental book entitled, ***Cancer: Its Causes, Symptoms and Treatment*** (1911). He was unique in that he practiced allopathy, homeopathy, Eclecticism, Physio-Medicalism, and Bio-chemic therapy each exclusively for five years (Jones, 1989). He developed a system of Definite Medication and really focused on the treatment of cancer.

Eli Jones' Paste No. 3

Therapeutic Principle

Escharotic.

Constituents

- 4 drams Solid extract bloodroot (*Sanguinaria canadensis*)
- 12 drams Zinc chloride
- 1 dram Starch
- 2 drams Red Saunders (*Pterocarpus santilinus*)

Form

Paste or salve.

Dosage
Apply as needed until tumor is gone.

Indication
Tumors, tumors of the breast, lip, hand, foot, arm or back, actinic keratosis, growths.

Application
Tumors, breast tumors, skin tumors, lip tumors, warts.

Contraindication
Only use under the supervision of a trained professional.

Herbs and Actions
Bloodroot acts an escharotic and anti-cancer herb. Zinc chloride acts as a healing agent to the skin. Starch acts as an ingredient to hold the herbs in a paste form. Red Saunders acts as an astringent.

Modifications
Red Clover can be added to increase the alterative effect. Galangal root can be added to increase the escharotic effect. Cayenne pepper can be added as a stimulant. Goldenseal can be substituted for Bloodroot to form John Pattison's Enucleating Paste.

Notes
This formula was used by Dr. Eli Jones, who wrote ***Cancer: Its Causes, Symptoms and Treatment*** (1911). He recommended it in cases of breast cancer, lip cancer, hand cancer, foot cancer, arm cancer, and back cancer. Dr. Jones would apply the pastes with adhesive strips in order to keep the escharotics off of healthy tissue. Dressings were changed daily and bathed until the patient sensed a dead, heavy weight, at which time he would switch to a poultice, such as one made of Slippery Elm, Flax Seed, Lobelia Seed, and Bayberry Bark until the growth would separate.

Trifolium Compound/Hoxsey Formula

Therapeutic Principle

Blood purifier; invigorate the circulation; lymphatic and glandular alterative.

Constituents

- 2 parts Red Clover Blossom (*Trifolium pratense*)
- 2 parts Licorice (*Glycyrriza glabra*)
- ½ part Buckthorn Bark (*Rhamnus frangula*)
- 1 part Burdock (*Arctium lappa*)
- 1 part Stillingia Root (*Stillingia sylvatica*)
- 1 part Oregon Grape Root (*Berberis aquifolium*)
- ½ part Phytolacca Root (*Phytolacca americana*)
- ½ part Prickly Ash Bark (*Xanthoxylum clava-herculis*)
- 1/8 part Wild Indigo Root (*Baptisia tinctoria*)
- Potassium Iodide USP

Form

Decoction.

Dosage

Tea, three cups per day warm. Tincture, 30-60 drops three times per day.

Indication

Pain of a fixed nature, anorexia, wasting, glandular swelling, glandular congestion, loss of voice, sore throat, constipation, sinus pain and congestion, joint pain, pain in the ear, and moist, red, irritable skin, irritability. The pulse tends to be wiry, taut, and hesitant, while the tongue usually appears dark red with purple spots. The lymphatic rosary and radii solaris can be present in the iris.

Application

Cancer, tumors, swollen lymph nodes, sore throat, constipation, laryngitis, bronchitis, pharyngitis, arthritis, skin diseases, chronic middle ear infections, detoxification.

Contraindication
Contraindicated in pregnancy and nursing mothers. Not to be taken for acute conditions associated with fever, inflammation, or infection (Smith, 1997).

Herbs and Actions
The herbs in this formula act as alteratives and blood purifiers. The formula's action is through the lymphatic, glandular and mucus membrane system, where it acts to alter disordered processes of the metabolic and catabolic humors, especially the elimination of metabolic waste (Smith, 1997). Red clover acts as an alterative and anti-cancer herb. Licorice acts as a demulcent and harmonizer. Buckthorn acts as a laxative. Burdock acts as an alterative, diaphoretic, and laxative. Stillingia acts as an alterative, with particular action on secretory and lymphatic functions, and is also anti-cancer. Oregon Grape Root acts as an alterative, lymphgogue, and anti-cancer herb. Prickly Ash acts as an alterative, tonic, and diaphoretic. Potassium iodide acts as an alterative and diuretic.

Modification
For amenorrhea and dysmenorrhea, add Mother's wort, Licorice, and Corydalis. For prostate cancer, add Saw Palmetto. For breast cancer, add Sheep Sorrel, Echinacea, and drop doses of Conium. Podophyllum can be added for more lymphatic work. Cascara can be added for a more purging action.

Commentary
The Trifolium Compound/Hoxsey formula is a very popular and time proven remedy for some cancers. Many patients have made successful trips to the Hoxsey clinic in Mexico. Trifolium Compound was first recorded by Parke, Davis & Co. in 1890. It was considered one of the most valuable alteratives known, indicated for skin disorders, scrofulosis, and syphilis, and used as a tonic to the excretory, assimilative, and digestive organs. King's American Dispensatory listed it in 1898 as a tonic, alterative, and eliminative used for scrofula, chronic rheumatism, syphilis, and glandular and skin conditions (King, 1989). Harry Hoxsey made the formula famous by using it quite successfully with many cancers.

Essiac Tea

Therapeutic Principle
Invigorate the blood circulation and remove blood stasis.

Constituents
- 52 parts Burdock Root (*Arctium lappa*)
- 16 parts Sheep Sorrel (*Rumex acetosella*)
- 1 part Turkey Rhubarb (*Rheum palmatum*)
- 4 parts Slippery Elm (*Ulmus fulva*)

Form
Decoction.

Dosage
Take four tablespoons or two ounces once in the morning, five minutes before eating, and once in the evening, at least two hours after eating. As a preventative, take daily four tablespoons or two ounces at bedtime or on an empty stomach at least two hours after eating.

Indication
Pain, chronic pain of a fixed and piercing nature, abdominal pain, pain with hardening, lumps, irritability, indigestion, constipation, insomnia, emotional upset. The tongue tends to be purple with spots on the side or dark red with purple spots. The pulse is usually wiry and taut, with a hesitancy. The lymphatic rosary and radii solaris can be present in the iris.

Application
Detoxification, cancer, AIDS, chronic fatigue, lupus, alzheimers, multiple sclerosis, chronic pain, coronary heart disease, tumors, anorexia.

Contraindication
Contraindicated in pregnancy.

Herbs and Actions

Sheep Sorrel and Burdock are the emperor herbs that act to destroy cancer. The Slippery Elm and Rhubarb assist by increasing bile flow and assisting the intestinal tract to eliminate the toxins released by the formula (Percival, 1994).

Modification

There is an optional modification of the formula, where is added 2 parts Kelp, 1 part Red Clover, 1 part Blessed Thistle, and 0.4 parts Watercress. This tends to enhance the effectiveness of the formula if directed to the thyroid gland and liver detoxification and blood purification (Percival, 1994).

Commentary

This very popular formula for cancer was handed down by an Ojibway herbalist to Rene Caisse (Essiac is Caisse spelled backwards), a Canadian nurse who treated many terminal cancer patients successfully.

Bibliography

Bergner, Paul; *Pharmacy Gems from William Cook*; Lecture at Pacific Northwest Herbal Symposium, Wilsonville, OR, 1999.

Bergner, Paul; ***Medical Herbalism: A Journal for the Clinical Practitioner***; Boulder, CO, 1997-2002.

Boyle, Wade, and Andre Saine; **Lectures in Naturopathic Hydrotherapy**; Buckeye Naturopathic Press, East Palestine, Ohio, 1988.

Boyle, Wade; *The History of Naturopathic Botanical Medicine*; Lecture at Gaia Herbal Symposium, Welches, OR, 1993.

Brinker, Francis J.; *The Hoxsey Treatment: Cancer Quackery or Effective Physiological Adjuvant?*, **Journal Of Naturopathic Medicine**, Vol. 6, No. 1, Norwalk, CT, 1996.

Chiltoskey, Mary, and Paul Hamel; **Cherokee Plants: Their Uses- A 400 Year History**; Cherokee, NC, 1975.

Christopher, John R.; **School of Natural Healing**; Christopher Publications, Springville, Utah, 1996.

Clymer, R. Swinburne; **The Medicines of Nature: The Thomsonian System**; The Humanitarian Society, Quakertown, PA, 1905.

Colby, Benjamin; **A Guide to Health, Being an Exposition of the Thomsonian System of Practice**; John Burns, Milford, NH, 1846.

Cook, William; **The Physio-Medical Dispensatory: A Treatise on Therapeutics, Materia Medica, and Pharmacy in Accordance with the Principles of Physiological Medication**; Eclectic Medical Publications, Portland, OR, 1985, (1849).

Culpeper, Nicholas; **Culpeper's Complete Herbal**; Wordsworth Editions Ltd, Hertfordshire, England, 1995, (1653).

Dean, C.B.; **Domestic Medicine**; Hudson-Kimberly Publishing Company, Kansas City, MO, 1903.

Deschauer, Thomas; **Complete Course in Herbalism**; Thomas Deschauer, 1940.

Doane, Nancy Locke; **Indian Doctor Book**; Aerial Photography Services, Inc., Charlotte, NC.

Dominion Herbal College; **Master Herbology**; Dominion Herbal College Ltd., Vancouver, British Columbia, Canada, 1926.

Ehret, Arnold; **Mucusless Diet Healing System**; Benedict Lust Publications, New York, NY, 1970.

Ellingwood, Finley; **American Materia Medica, Therapeutics, and Pharmacognosy**; Eclectic Medical Publications, Portland, OR, 1985.

Felter, Harvey Wickes; **The Eclectic Materia Medica, Pharmacology, and Therapeutics**; John K. Scudder, Cincinnati, Ohio, 1922.

Felter, Harvey Wickes, and John Uri Lloyd; **King's American Dispensatory, Volumes I and II**; Eclectic Medical Publications, Portland, OR, 1983.

Fruehauf, Heiner, and Subhuti Dharmananda; **Pearls from the Golden Cabinet: The Practitioner's Guide to the Use of Chinese Herbs and Traditional Formulas**; Institute for Traditional Medicine, Portland, OR, 1993.

Griggs, Barbara; **Green Pharmacy: The History and Evolution of Western Herbal Medicine**; Healing Arts Press, Rochester, VT, 1981.

Jacobs, Thad, and Chris Meletis; **Interactions Between Drugs and Natural Medicines: What the Physician and Pharmacist Must Know About Vitamins, Minerals, Foods and Herbs**; Eclectic Medical Publications, Sandy, OR, 1999.

Jones, Eli; **Reading the Eye, Pulse, and Tongue for the Indicated Remedy**; Buckeye Naturopathic Press, East Palestine, OH, 1989.

Jones, Eli G.; **Cancer: Its Causes, Symptoms and Treatment**; B. Jain Publishers, New Delhi, India, 1994.

Kloss, Jethro; **Back to Eden**; Back to Eden Books Publishing Company, Loma Linda, CA, 1939.

Kneipp, Sebastian; **My Water Cure**; Thorsons Publishers Limited, Wellingborough, Northhamptonshire, England, 1979,(1893).

Kuts-Cheraux, A.W.; **Naturae Medicina and Naturopathic Dispensatory**; American Naturopathic Physicians and Surgeons Association, Des Moines, IA, 1953,

Lust, John; **The Herb Book**; Bantam Books, New York, NY, 1974.

Lyle, T.J.; **Physio-Medical Therapeutics, Materia Medica, and Pharmacy**; The National Association of Medical Herbalist of Great Britain, Ltd., London, England, 1932, (1897).

Meyer, Joseph; **The Herbalist**; Hammond Book Company, Hammond, IN, 1934.

Meyer, Joseph; **The Old Herb Doctor**; Hammond Book Company, Hammond, IN, 1941.

Mitchell, William A.; **Plant Medicine: Applications of the Botanical Remedies in the Practice of Naturopathic Medicine**; Preparatory Manuscript, 2000.

Mooney, James; **The Sacred Formulas of the Cherokees**; Bureau of American Ethnology, 1891.

Moore, Lawrence Emory; Oral Transmission and Apprenticeship, the Southern United States, 1963-1999.

Moss, Ralph W.; **Herbs Against Cancer: History and Controversy**; Equinox Press, Brooklyn, NY, 1998.

Naiman, Ingrid; **Cancer Salves: A Botanical Approach to Treatment**; Seventh Ray Press, Santa Fe, NM, 1999.

Percival, James; **The Essiac Handbook**; Rideout Publishing Company, Orlando, FL, 1994.

Priest, A.W., and L.R. Priest; **Herbal Medication: A Clinical and Dispensary Handbook**; L.N. Fowler and Company Ltd., London, England, 1982.

Rauch, Erich; **Naturopathic Treatment of Colds and Infectious Diseases**; Haug International, Brussels, Belgium, 1993,(1967).

Scudder, John M.; **Specific Diagnosis**; Eclectic Medicine Press, Sandy, OR, 1994.

Sherman, John A.; **The Complete Botanical Prescriber**; 1993.

Shook, Edward E.; **Advanced Treatise in Herbology**; Trinity Center Press, Beaumont, CA, 1978.

Simmonite, William Joseph; **The Simmonite-Culpeper Herbal Remedies**; W. Foulsham and Company Ltd., London, England, 1957.

Smith, Ed; **Therapeutic Herb Manual: The Therapeutic Administration of Medicinal Herb Compounds**; Ed Smith, Williams, OR, 1997.

Stamets, Zeanith H.; **Botanical Research and Treatment of Disease**; Z.H. Stamets, Fort Wayne, IN, 1954.

Strehlow, Wighard, and Gottfried Hertzka; **Hildegard of Bingen's Medicine**; Bear and Company, Santa Fe, NM, 1988.

Tierra, Michael; **Planetary Herbology**; Lotus Press, Twin Lakes, WI, 1988.

Tobyn, Graeme; **Culpeper's Medicine: A Practice of Western Holistic Medicine**; Element, Rockport, MA, 1997.

Weiss, Rudolf Fritz; **Herbal Medicine**; Beaconsfield Publishers, LTD, Beaconsfield, England, 1988.

Wren, R.C.; **Potter's New Cyclopaedia of Botanical Drugs and Preparations**; C.W. Daniel Company Limited, Essex, England, 1988.

Yance, Donald R. Jr.; **Herbal Medicine, Healing and Cancer**; Keats Publishing, Chicago, IL, 1999.

Zhongjing, Zhang; **Shang Han Lun**; New World Press, Beijing, China, 1993.

Index

U

V

W